We're KILLING OUR KIDS WITHDRAWN

How to End the Epidemic of **Overweight & Sedentary Children**

TODD HOLLANDER

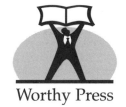

Worthy Press

www.worthypress.com

12 +0407

NOV ~ 9 2010

ATTENTION CORPORATIONS, UNIVERSITIES, COLLEGES, AND PROFESSIONAL ORGANIZATIONS: Quantity discounts are available for bulk purchases of this book for educational or gift purposes, and as premiums for increasing subscriptions or renewals. Special books or book excerpts can also be created to fit specific needs. For information, please contact:

Worthy Press
P.O. Box 888685
Atlanta, GA 30356
sales@worthypress.com
www.worthypress.com

Library of Congress Cataloging-in-Publication Data

Hollander, Todd
    We're killing our kids. How to end the epidemic of overweight and sedentary children / by Todd Hollander
        p. cm.
    Includes bibliographical references and index.
    ISBN 0-9753166-4-8

2004093458

10 9 8 7 6 5 4 3 2 1

Cover design by Susanne Van Duyne (Trade Design Group)
Cover image by Getty Images Inc.

To Amy, Ashley, and Parker. I wish I had known when you were younger what I know now. Thank you for your cheerfulness and enthusiasm in adopting a healthy lifestyle and helping to share the good news.

Table of Contents

List of Tables and Figures

About the Author

Todd Hollander is a market research consultant with 20 years experience designing and managing strategic research principally for Fortune 500 companies. His expertise includes research methodology, data collection, analysis, and strategic development. He serves as instructor in Principles of Marketing Research, University of Georgia. For more information see www.toddhollander.com.

Hollander has been married for 16 years. His twin teenage daughters and pre-teenage son are living examples of the effectiveness of the concepts and strategy presented in *We're Killing Our Kids*.

How to Contact

Todd Hollander
c/o Worthy Press
PO Box 888685
Atlanta, GA 30356

"The first wealth is health."
— *Ralph Waldo Emerson*

INTRODUCTION

ഓരലഓരലഓരലഓരലഓരലഓരലഓരലഓരലഓരലഓരലഓരലഓരലഓരല

"Our nation's young people are, in large measure, inactive, unfit, and increasingly overweight. In the long run, this physical inactivity threatens to reverse the decades-long progress we have made in reducing death from cardiovascular diseases and to devastate our national health care budget. In the short run, physical inactivity has contributed to an unprecedented epidemic of childhood obesity that is currently plaguing the United States."

- Report to the President from the Secretary of Health and Human Services and the Secretary of Education, Fall 2000

ഓരലഓരലഓരലഓരലഓരലഓരലഓരലഓരലഓരലഓരലഓരലഓരലഓരല

The children of America are the fattest children in the world. In the last 20 years, the prevalence of overweight American children has increased so dramatically that the American Academy of Pediatrics claims, "Overweight is now the most common medical condition of childhood."[1] Once a rare affliction, childhood obesity has become so pervasive that it is

11

commonly referred to as an *epidemic* – a word that is not used lightly in the healthcare community.

Today, more than 30 percent of Americans ages 6-19 are overweight, and at least 15 percent are obese.[2] This means that in a group of only seven children, the odds are that one is overweight and another is obese. Since 1976, the prevalence of obesity has doubled for children ages 6-11 and tripled for adolescents ages 12-19. As these young people age, their poor eating habits and sedentary lifestyles will cause not only an unprecedented rate of premature death and disability, but also serious financial repercussions for their families, insurers, and healthcare providers.

This book is both a call to action and a guidebook. It is intended to help parents, grandparents, educators, caregivers, and other concerned adults understand:

- How to objectively assess a child's weight.
- The ten leading causes of this epidemic.
- The consequences of poor nutrition and sedentary lifestyles.
- The myths and facts about nutrition, exercise, and weight loss.
- How to help children eat properly and get plenty of exercise.

The book is based not only on extensive research but also on personal experience. Like millions of Americans, I spent the better part of my adult life with a weight problem. Like many, I allowed the demands of work, family, and community to supercede physical fitness. Although I followed the food guide pyramid and fastidiously avoided dietary fat, I approached my 40th birthday 30 pounds overweight and suffering from high blood pressure, high cholesterol, and high triglycerides. Aware that these conditions dramatically increased my risk for premature death or disability, I made a commitment to solving my weight problem.

I joined a gym and after several months had succeeded in dropping a few pounds, but my blood pressure, cholesterol, and triglycerides remained elevated. Frustrated, I decided to conduct some research. After all, I was a professional market researcher. If I could help some of the nation's most successful companies solve their problems, surely I could apply the same skills to discover why a low-fat diet was not helping me lose weight.

I started my research by reading about nutrition. What I learned was both shocking and liberating. It became clear that the low-fat, high-carbohydrate diet was not only incapable of solving my weight problem—it seemed to be *causing* it.

As a result of this revelation, I focused my nutritional research on alternatives to the low-fat, high-carbohydrate diet, one of which was the Zone diet advocated by Dr. Barry Sears.[3] This approach to weight loss was based on using foods to balance hormone and insulin levels. Sears claimed that eating the right foods in the right combinations at the right times would result in permanent weight loss and enhanced physical and mental performance (what athletes call being "in the zone"). After discussing the program with several people who had used it to achieve lasting results, I decided to give it a try. The Zone diet worked for me, but not as well as I had hoped. After a couple of months, I had lost a few more pounds but seemed to have hit a wall. Try as I might, I could not lose any more weight.

One day I bumped into an old friend and noticed that he had lost a considerable amount of weight. When I asked how he did it, he told me he had been on the Sugar Busters diet and explained that the Sugar Busters approach is to decrease consumption of "bad carbohydrates" (corn, potatoes, processed grains, refined sugar, and white rice) and increase consumption of "good carbohydrates" (fruits, high fiber vegetables, and whole grains). The next day I picked up a copy of *Sugar Busters! Cut Sugar to Trim Fat.*[4] I began following the book's recommendations and embarked on a way of eating that, combined with daily exercise, helped me to lose over 25 pounds, reduce my cholesterol, and lower my blood pressure.

With my newfound knowledge about carbohydrates, I began to see the world through different eyes. One of the things I saw shocked me. As I looked at my three children, I recognized that with the best of intentions my wife and I had been serving them meals and snacks that were virtually guaranteed to make them overweight. Compounding this problem was the fact that we had allowed their lives to become increasingly sedentary. In short, I realized that we were killing our kids. The remedy was not only to change the children's diet but also to increase their physical activity. To avoid resistance or outright mutiny, I knew we needed a plan. I also knew that developing an effective plan would require additional research. *We're Killing Our Kids* is the result of that research and the experience of applying it to my family.

I have taken the same approach to this book that I have used to serve many of the nation's most successful corporations: collect and analyze data, identify implications, and develop appropriate actions. I do not presume to have all the answers, but of this I am certain: Our children are sick and we must take immediate action to help them. It is my sincere desire that this book will provide you the information, tools, and motivation to help children develop lifelong habits of healthy eating and physical fitness.

Overweight and Obesity: Measurements, Definitions, and Statistics

ഇൻ Cൻ ഇൻ Cൻ ഇൻ Cൻ ഇൻ Cൻ ഇൻ Cൻ ഇൻ Cൻ

"A problem clearly stated is a
problem half solved."

– *Dorothea Brande*

ഇൻ Cൻ ഇൻ Cൻ ഇൻ Cൻ ഇൻ Cൻ ഇൻ Cൻ ഇൻ Cൻ

Part 1. Measurements

Body Mass Index

The most common way to determine if a child is overweight is to use a calculation called *Body Mass Index (BMI)*. Calculating BMI requires only two pieces of data–weight and height–which can be measured either in pounds and inches or kilograms and meters. The following formulas are used to calculate BMI.

Body Mass Index (BMI) Calculations

English Formula

$$BMI = \frac{\text{Weight in Pounds}}{\text{Height in Inches}^2} \times 703$$

Metric Formula

$$BMI = \frac{\text{Weight in Kilograms}}{\text{Height in Meters}^2}$$

or

$$\frac{\text{Weight in Kilograms}}{\text{Height in Centimeters}^2} \times 10,000$$

Advantages

One advantage of using BMI is its simplicity. Because it is such an easy formula, BMI can be calculated for children all over the world. Additionally, because it takes height into account, BMI is a more accurate reflection of body fat content than the traditional weight-for-age approach.

Disadvantages

For most people, BMI is a reliable indicator of total body fat content.[1] However, because BMI does not account for body composition, which includes the proportions of muscle, bone, fat, and other tissues that constitute a person's total body weight, it can sometimes overestimate or underestimate body fat. For example, BMI may:

- **Overestimate** body fat in athletes and others who have a muscular build. Such individuals may have a BMI that is considered overweight or obese even though they may have little body fat.

- **Underestimate** body fat in the elderly and others who have lost muscle mass. Such people may have a normal BMI when in fact they actually have too much body fat.

Critics of BMI generally recommend more accurate measurements of body fat content such as waist-to-hip measurements, waist circumference, underwater weighing, or skin caliper testing. Although these methods may be more accurate than simple BMI calculations, the fact that they require special equipment or training makes their widespread use impractical. Thus, while BMI is not a perfect tool, it is the best tool currently available to assess the weight of large numbers of people, especially children.

BMI Diary-Entry #1

Appendix A includes a Body Mass Index Diary that will enable you to track your child's progress in reducing BMI (this tool can also be downloaded free of charge from www.worthypress.com/wkok/diary.htm). The first thing to record in this diary is the current BMI for each child age two or older. To use the table, find the child's height in the left-hand column of page 21 or 22. Move across to the child's current weight. The number at the top of the column is the BMI at that height and weight. Please take a moment to look up each child's BMI in Table 1 and record it in the diary.

Table 1
Body Mass Index for Children

BMI / Height (inches)	13	14	15	16	17	18	19	20	21	22	23	24	25	26	27	28	29	30	31	32	33	34	35	36
								Body Weight (pounds)																
33	20	21	23	24	26	27	29	30	32	34	35	37	38	40	41	43	44	46	48	49	51	52	54	55
34	21	23	24	26	27	29	31	32	34	36	37	39	41	42	44	46	47	49	50	52	54	55	57	59
35	22	24	26	27	29	31	33	34	36	38	40	41	43	45	47	48	50	52	54	55	57	59	60	62
36	23	25	27	29	31	33	35	36	38	40	42	44	46	47	49	51	53	55	57	58	60	62	64	66
37	25	27	29	31	33	35	37	38	40	42	44	46	48	50	52	54	56	58	60	62	64	66	68	70
38	26	28	30	32	34	36	39	41	43	45	47	49	51	53	55	57	59	61	63	65	67	69	71	73
39	28	30	32	34	36	38	41	43	45	47	49	51	54	56	58	60	62	64	67	69	71	73	75	77
40	29	31	34	36	38	40	43	45	47	50	52	54	56	59	61	63	66	68	70	72	75	77	79	81
41	31	33	35	38	40	42	45	47	50	52	54	57	59	62	64	66	69	71	74	76	78	81	83	86
42	32	35	37	40	42	45	47	50	52	55	57	60	62	65	67	70	72	75	77	80	82	85	87	90
43	34	36	39	42	44	47	49	52	55	57	60	63	65	68	71	73	76	78	81	84	86	89	92	94
44	35	38	41	44	46	49	52	55	57	60	63	66	68	71	74	77	79	82	85	88	90	93	96	99
45	37	40	43	46	48	51	54	57	60	63	66	69	72	74	77	80	83	86	89	92	95	97	100	103
46	39	42	45	48	51	54	57	60	63	66	69	72	75	78	81	84	87	90	93	96	99	102	105	108
47	40	43	47	50	53	56	59	62	65	69	72	75	78	81	84	87	91	94	97	100	103	106	109	113
48	42	45	49	52	55	58	62	65	68	72	75	78	81	85	88	91	95	98	101	104	108	111	114	117
49	44	47	51	54	58	61	64	68	71	75	78	81	85	88	92	95	99	102	105	109	112	116	119	122
50	46	49	53	56	60	64	67	71	74	78	81	85	88	92	96	99	103	106	110	113	117	120	124	128
51	48	51	55	59	62	66	70	73	77	81	85	88	92	96	99	103	107	110	114	118	122	125	129	133
52	50	53	57	61	65	69	73	76	80	84	88	92	96	100	103	107	111	115	119	123	126	130	134	138
53	51	55	59	63	67	71	75	79	83	87	91	95	99	103	107	111	115	119	123	127	131	135	139	143
54	53	58	62	66	70	74	78	82	87	91	95	99	103	107	111	116	120	124	128	132	136	141	145	149
55	55	60	64	68	73	77	81	86	90	94	98	103	107	111	116	120	124	129	133	137	141	146	150	154

To use the table, find the child's height in the left-hand column of this page or the next. Move across to the current weight. The number at the top of the column is the BMI at that height and weight.

Body Mass Index for Children

BMI Height (inches)	13	14	15	16	17	18	19	20	21	22	23	24	25	26	27	28	29	30	31	32	33	34	35	36
											Body Weight (pounds)													
56	57	62	66	71	75	80	84	89	93	98	102	107	111	115	120	124	129	133	138	142	147	151	156	160
57	60	64	69	73	78	83	87	92	97	101	106	110	115	120	124	129	134	138	143	147	152	157	161	166
58	62	66	71	76	81	86	90	95	100	105	110	114	119	124	129	133	138	143	148	153	157	162	167	172
59	64	69	74	79	84	89	94	99	103	108	113	118	123	128	133	138	143	148	153	158	163	168	173	178
60	66	71	76	81	87	92	97	102	107	112	117	122	128	133	138	143	148	153	158	163	168	174	179	184
61	68	74	79	84	89	95	100	105	111	116	121	127	132	137	142	148	153	158	164	169	174	179	185	190
62	71	76	82	87	92	98	103	109	114	120	125	131	136	142	147	153	158	164	169	174	180	185	191	196
63	73	79	84	90	95	101	107	112	118	124	129	135	141	146	152	158	163	169	175	180	186	191	197	203
64	75	81	87	93	99	104	110	116	122	128	134	139	145	151	157	163	169	174	180	186	192	198	203	209
65	78	84	90	96	102	108	114	120	126	132	138	144	150	156	162	168	174	180	186	192	198	204	210	216
66	80	86	92	99	105	111	117	123	130	136	142	148	154	161	167	173	179	185	192	198	204	210	216	223
67	83	89	95	102	108	114	121	127	134	140	146	153	159	166	172	178	185	191	197	204	210	217	223	229
68	85	92	98	105	111	118	124	131	138	144	151	157	164	171	177	184	190	197	203	210	217	223	230	236
69	88	94	101	108	115	121	128	135	142	148	155	162	169	176	182	189	196	203	209	216	223	230	237	243
70	90	97	104	111	118	125	132	139	146	153	160	167	174	181	188	195	202	209	216	223	230	236	243	250
71	93	100	107	114	121	129	136	143	150	157	164	172	179	186	193	200	207	215	222	229	236	243	250	258
72	95	103	110	117	125	132	140	147	154	162	169	176	184	191	199	206	213	221	228	235	243	250	258	265
73	98	106	113	121	128	136	144	151	159	166	174	181	189	197	204	212	219	227	234	242	250	257	265	272
74	101	109	116	124	132	140	148	155	163	171	179	186	194	202	210	218	225	233	241	249	257	264	272	280
75	104	112	120	128	136	144	152	160	168	176	184	192	200	208	216	224	232	240	248	256	264	272	280	288
76	106	115	123	131	139	147	156	164	172	180	188	197	205	213	221	230	238	246	254	262	271	279	287	295
77	109	118	126	134	143	151	160	168	177	185	193	202	210	219	227	236	244	253	261	269	278	286	295	303
78	112	121	129	138	147	155	164	173	181	190	199	207	216	225	233	242	250	259	268	276	285	294	302	311

Part 2: Definitions

Having recorded the current BMI of each child, the next step is to assess what these numbers mean.

BMI Classifications

BMI classifications for children are determined by using special growth charts developed by the Centers for Disease Control and Prevention (CDC). The CDC charts are age-specific because body composition changes over the growth period. They are also gender-specific because boys and girls differ in body composition as they mature.

The following figures show the BMI-for-age percentiles for boys (Figure 1) and girls (Figure 2) ages 2 to 20. On these charts, the 5th, 10th, 25th, 50th, 75th, 85th, 90th, and 95th percentiles for BMI are plotted for each age.

Figure 1

CDC Growth Charts: United States

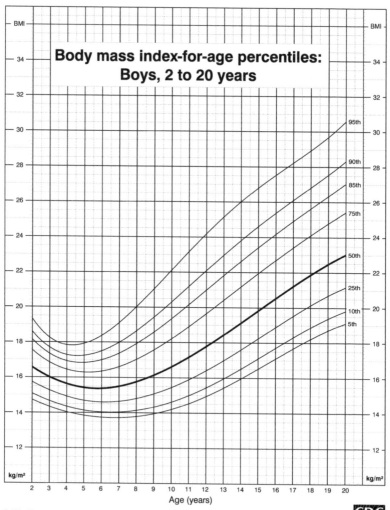

Body mass index-for-age percentiles: Boys, 2 to 20 years

Published May 30, 2000.
SOURCE: Developed by the National Center for Health Statistics in collaboration with the National Center for Chronic Disease Prevention and Health Promotion (2000).

CDC
SAFER · HEALTHIER · PEOPLE™

Figure 2

CDC Growth Charts: United States

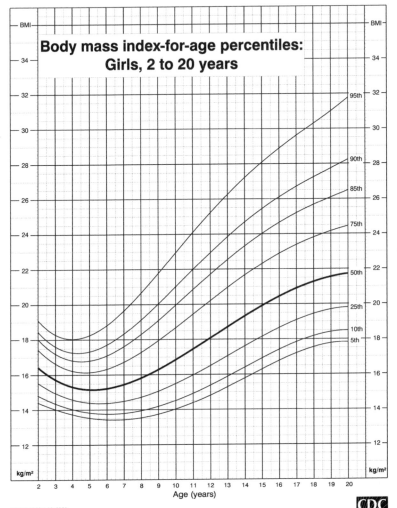

Body mass index-for-age percentiles: Girls, 2 to 20 years

Published May 30, 2000.
SOURCE: Developed by the National Center for Health Statistics in collaboration with
the National Center for Chronic Disease Prevention and Health Promotion (2000).

CDC
SAFER·HEALTHIER·PEOPLE™

The American Obesity Association (AOA) defines children and adolescents at or above the 85th percentile as *overweight*,[2] which corresponds to an adult BMI of 25. The AOA uses the 95th percentile as the threshold of childhood obesity because it:

- Corresponds to an adult BMI of 30, which is the threshold for adult obesity.

- Is associated with elevated blood pressure and lipids in older adolescents, and increases their risk of diseases.

- Identifies children whose obesity is likely to persist into adulthood.

- Is recommended as a marker for when children and adolescents should have in-depth medical assessments.

- Is a criterion in clinical trials of childhood obesity treatments.

- Is a criterion for more aggressive treatment.

Unlike the American Obesity Association, some groups make no distinction between overweight and obesity. Instead, they simply refer to any child at or above the 95th percentile as being overweight. Because this practice dramatically understates the prevalence of overweight children, the statistics presented in the following section adhere to the AOA definitions.

BMI Diary-Entry #2

Having gained an understanding of what the BMI numbers mean, the next step is to record the percentile for each child in the Body Mass Index Diary (Appendix A). Use either the chart for boys on page 24 or the chart for girls on page 25. Plot the child's age on the horizontal axis. Next, on the vertical axis, plot the BMI previously obtained from Table 1 on pages 21 and 22. Finally, identify the BMI percentile by moving up to the next curve. For example, in Figure 1, a 12-year-old boy with a BMI of 20 falls in the 85th percentile; a 13-year-old boy with a BMI of 20 is in the 75th percentile.

Important Note

If your child's BMI falls lower than the 85th percentile, breathe a sigh of relief, but do not stop reading. The information in the following chapters will help you ensure that your child maintains a healthy weight through proper nutrition and regular exercise.

Part 3: Statistics

In 1999, the CDC published the following list of the most significant public health achievements of the past 100 years.[3]

Top 10 U.S. Public Health Achievements of the 20ᵗʰ Century

- Vaccination

- Motor-vehicle safety

- Safer workplaces

- Control of infectious diseases

- Decline in deaths from coronary heart disease and stroke

- Safer and healthier foods

- Healthier mothers and babies

- Family planning

- Fluoridation of drinking water

- Recognition of tobacco use as a health hazard

Source: Centers for Disease Control and Prevention (CDC)

As this list demonstrates, the twentieth century produced unprecedented improvements in the health of Americans. During this period, infant mortality decreased by 90 percent and life expectancy increased by 30 years.[4] In the second half of the

> *30% of*
>
> *Americans*
>
> *ages 6-19 are*
>
> *overweight;*
>
> *15% are obese.*

century, age-adjusted death rates from cardiovascular disease declined 60 percent, representing one of the most important public health achievements in the nation's history. This is the good news.

The bad news is that our children are part of an epidemic of overweight and obesity that, if left unchecked, is likely to undo many of the public health advances achieved during the last century. According to data from the CDC, 30 percent of Americans ages 6-19 are overweight, and 15 percent are obese.[5] This means that over 17 million 6-19 year-olds are overweight and at least 8.6 million are obese.[5, 6] Even preschoolers are included in this epidemic, with over 20 percent of children ages 2-5 overweight and at least 10 percent obese.[5]

Among children and adolescents, the problem of overweight and obesity affects both genders and every racial, ethnic, and age group.[5] In the last 20 years, the prevalence of overweight American children has increased so dramatically that the American Academy of Pediatrics has asserted, "Overweight is now the most common medical condition of childhood."[7]

As a professional market researcher, I know that statistics often tell a story. Consider the information in Table 2. In 1963, the year in which I was born, only four percent of children and five percent of adolescents were obese. By the time I graduated from high school in 1981, obesity among children had ticked up to seven percent. At this point, something dramatic started to happen. During the period between my wedding (1988) and the birth of our children (1990-1995), the percentage of obese children and adolescents rose dramatically to a total of 11 percent. By the time my last child started kindergarten (2000), the incidence of obese children and adolescents had risen to an alarming 15 percent.

Table 2

Prevalence of Obese Children and Adolescents

Age	1963-70	1971-74	1976-80	1988-94	1999-2000
6-11	4	4	7	11	15
12-19	5	6	5	11	15

Source: CDC, National Health and Nutrition Examination Surveys (NHANES) 1976-2000

In short, the percentage of obese children and adolescents has tripled in my lifetime. If the trend continues, this is likely to be the first generation of Americans with a shorter natural lifespan than the preceding generation. While immediate and effective action is clearly called for, the first step toward reversing the epidemic of childhood overweight is to understand what is causing it.

> **If the trend continues, this is likely to be the first generation of Americans with a shorter natural lifespan than the preceding generation.**

2

Causes

CR80CR80CR80CR80CR CR CR CR CR80CR80CR80CR80CR
"Where the cause is not known the
effect cannot be produced."
— *Francis Bacon*
CR80CR80CR80CR80CR CR CR CR CR80CR80CR80CR80CR

Cause 1. Society

Times have changed. For most of the nation's history, overweight children were rare. In the "good old days," there were no computers, video games, cable television, or fast food restaurants. Children walked to and from school, often a distance of several miles (though not, as many a grandparent has claimed, uphill in both directions). They did daily chores that demanded considerable physical exertion. Playtime involved riding bicycles, climbing trees, and playing "Tag," "Hide and Seek" and "Kick the Can." Most meals were prepared and eaten at home.

Today, Americans drive more and walk less. According to the 2001 Department of Transportation

33

National Household Travel Survey[1], the number of "walking trips" Americans make on a typical day has declined by 40 percent since 1977. As a result, 90 percent of all trips made by adults and 70 percent of all trips made by children are now made in automobiles. Children's walking trips have declined 60 percent since 1977, and walking and bicycling trips to school have declined 50 percent since 1969. This decline is due in part to the increase in traffic and crime, which have rendered many streets too dangerous for children to walk or bike to school.

> **Everyday life has ceased to require the physical exertion necessary to maintain healthy weight and physical fitness.**

Longer school days and increased participation in after-school activities have resulted in significantly less time for household chores or outdoor play. The dramatic rise in both parents working has left little time for either to prepare meals at home. Consequently, the proportion of meals eaten in restaurants and fast food establishments has increased significantly. With the decline of the family farm and the invention of new technologies, everyday life has ceased to require the physical exertion necessary to maintain healthy weight and physical fitness. All of these changes have helped create an environment conducive to overweight and obesity.

Cause 2. Innovation

As shown in the following table, the 20th century produced numerous innovations, many of which have dramatically improved the quality of life in America. Some of these innovations, such as the escalator, color television, personal computer, and the Internet, have had the unintended effect of decreasing children's physical activity. Others, including frozen pizza and fast food restaurants, have increased food consumption. Many of these innovations have contributed to the epidemic of childhood overweight and obesity.

Table 3

20th Century Innovations

Year	Innovation	Year	Innovation	Year	Innovation
1900	Escalator	1943	Synthetic Rubber		Arpanet (First Internet)
1901	Disk Brakes	1946	Microwave Oven	1969	Automatic Teller Machine
	Radio Receiver	1947	Transistor		Bar-Code Scanner
	Telegraph		Tupperware		Wendy's
	Vacuum Cleaner	1948	Frisbee	1970	Daisy-Wheel Printer
1903	Bottle-Making Machinery		Jukebox		Floppy Disk
	Airplane	1949	Cake Mix		Dot-Matrix Printer
1904	Tractor	1951	Power Steering		Food Processor
	Vacuum Tube		Videotape Recorder	1971	Liquid-Crystal Display (LCD)
1907	Bakelite Cookware	1952	Diet Soft Drink		Microprocessor
	Helicopter		Kentucky Fried Chicken		VCR
1908	Cellophane	1953	Frozen Pizza		Video Disc
	Model T		Transistor Radio	1972	Video Game
1909	Instant Coffee		Nonstick Pan		Word Processor
1910	Talking Motion Picture	1954	Solar Cell	1973	Ethernet Computer Network
1911	Automobile Electric Ignition		McDonalds	1974	Post-It Note
1915	Pyrex		Burger King	1975	Laser Printer
1916	Radio Tuner	1955	Optic Fiber	1976	Ink-Jet Printer
	Stainless Steel		Computer Hard Disk	1978	Spreadsheet Software
1919	Pop-Up Toaster	1956	Hovercraft		Cellular Phones
	Short-Wave Radio		Liquid Paper	1979	Cray Supercomputer
	Traffic Signal	1957	Fortran Computer Language		Walkman
1923	Cathode-Ray Tube		Modem		Roller Blades
	Self-Winding Watch	1958	Laser	1981	MS-DOS
	Birdseye Frozen Food		Integrated Circuit		Personal Computer
1928	Electric Shaver		Pizza Hut	1983	Apple Lisa Computer
	Bubble Gum	1959	Microchip		Compact Disc Player
1933	Electric Dishwasher		Denny's	1984	CD-ROM
1933	FM Radio	1960	Domino's		Apple Macintosh Computer
	Stereo Records		Audio Cassette	1985	Windows Operating System
1934	Tape Recorder	1962	Computer Video Game	1986	Super-Conductor
1935	Canned Beer		Taco Bell	1987	3-D Video Game
1937	Photocopier		Permanent-Press Fabric	1988	Digital Cellular Phones
	Jet Engine	1964	BASIC Computer Language	1989	High-Definition Television
	Freeze-Dried Coffee		Blimpie	1990	World Wide Web
1938	Teflon		Astroturf	1991	Digital Answering Machine
	Turboprop Engine	1965	Nutrasweet	1993	Pentium Processor
1939	Electron Microscope		Subway		
	Helicopter	1966	Electronic Fuel Injection		
1940	Color Television	1967	Handheld Calculator		
	Dairy Queen	1968	Computer Mouse		
1941	Aerosol Spray Cans		Random Access Memory		

Cause 3. Electronic Media

There is no doubt about it: Kids today watch a lot of television. Table 4 shows the results of a study conducted by Nielsen Media Research[2] that revealed the following.

Table 4
Television Ownership and Use

- Virtually every household in America has a television; 34% have two; 41% have three or more.

- In the average American home, the television is on for over seven hours per day.

- 49% of Americans say they watch too much TV.

- Children ages 2-11 watch an average of 20 hours of television per week.

- American children watch television an average of 1,023 hours per year (compared to only 900 hours per year spent in school).

- The odds that an American parent requires children to complete homework before watching television are 1 in 12.

- 73% of parents would like to limit the time their children spend watching television.

Source: Nielsen Media Research 2000

In the majority of American homes, children have access to 50 or more television channels as well as videotapes, DVDs, and video games. Research has shown that:

- 48% of all families with children ages 2-17 have all four of the media staples: TV, VCR, video game, and computer.[3]

- 57% of children ages 8-16 have a television in their bedrooms. [4]

- 6½ hours per day is the average time children spend using media.[5] (Figure 3)

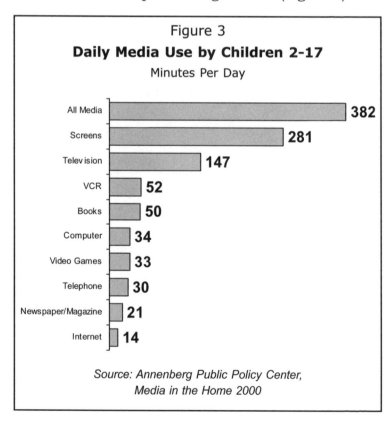

Figure 3
Daily Media Use by Children 2-17
Minutes Per Day

All Media	382
Screens	281
Television	147
VCR	52
Books	50
Computer	34
Video Games	33
Telephone	30
Newspaper/Magazine	21
Internet	14

*Source: Annenberg Public Policy Center,
Media in the Home 2000*

Prescbool Coucb Potatoes

A study conducted by the Kaiser Family Foundation[6] found that overindulgence in electronic media is not isolated to older children. This research revealed that children from six months to six years old spend an average of two hours a day (1:58) using screen media, about the same amount of time spent playing outside (2:01). Additional findings include:

> **There is a high correlation between television viewing and weight.**

- **Bedroom Media:** More than a third (36%) of children ages six and younger had televisions in their bedrooms; more than one quarter (27%) had VCRs or DVD players; one tenth had video game players; seven percent had a computer. Thirty percent of children ages three and younger and 43 percent of four to six year-olds had TVs in their bedrooms.

- **Computers:** On a typical day, more than one quarter (27%) of children ages 4-6 used a computer, spending an average of just over one hour (1:04) at the keyboard. More than a third (39%) of 4-6 year-olds used a computer several times a week or more; 37 percent in this age group could turn the computer on by themselves, and 40 percent could load a CD-ROM.

- **Heavy TV households:** Many children lived in homes where the television was an ever-present companion: two-thirds (65%) lived in homes where the TV was left on at least half the time, even if no one was watching; more than one third (36%) lived in homes where the TV was on "always" or "most of the time."

It should come as no surprise that there is a high correlation between television viewing and weight. Researchers have determined that the incidence of obesity is highest among children who watch television four or more hours per day and lowest among those who watch one hour or less per day.[7] In a study of preschoolers ages 1-4, a child's risk of being overweight was found to increase six percent for every hour of television watched per day. For children with a television in the bedroom, the odds of being overweight jumped an additional 31 percent for every hour watched. Preschool children with TVs in their bedrooms watched an additional 4.8 hours of television or videos every week. [8]

The more children watch television, the less likely they are to exercise and the more likely they are to be overweight. Dr. Robert Klesges, a researcher at Memphis State University, found that "children watching TV tend to burn fewer calories per minute – not only fewer than those engaged in active play, but also fewer than those who are reading or 'doing nothing' – in fact, almost as few as children who are sleeping."[9] Klesges found that the heavier a child is, the more serious the effect. While television viewing triggered a 12 percent drop in metabolism for children of normal weight, the metabolic rates of obese children declined an average of 16 percent.

> *Limiting screen time and removing televisions from bedrooms can be important first steps in leading children to a more physically active lifestyle.*

The implication is clear: children should watch less television and engage in more physically demanding activities. Although some would say that the solution is to eliminate television viewing altogether, for most families this is impractical. Thus, the issue is probably not *whether* to watch television but *which* and *how many* shows to watch. Limiting screen time and removing televisions from bedrooms can be important first steps in leading children to a more physically active lifestyle.

Video Game Junkies

Video gaming systems such as GameCube, Xbox, and PlayStation, while perhaps mildly less passive than television, are far more consuming and some would say addicting. Because it is not unusual for children to spend hours at a time on these activities, video games and physical fitness are often mutually exclusive. Thus, it appears that weaning children from video games is a difficult but essential task.

> *Weaning children from video games is a difficult but essential task.*

Cause 4. Government

The U.S. Department of Agriculture has been issuing dietary recommendations for over 100 years. The best-known and most widely-accepted was the low-fat, high-carbohydrate diet that it began advocating in the late 1970s and which culminated in the publication of the Food Guide Pyramid in 1992.

When the USDA published its first dietary recommendations in 1894, a number of vitamins and minerals had not even been discovered, and malnutrition was a far greater concern than overconsumption. During the first half of the 20th century, researchers determined ways to prevent nutritional deficiencies such as scurvy and beriberi, and recommended food policies such as fortifying salt with iodine and enriching flour with vitamin B.

By the end of World War II, the prevalence of heart disease in the U.S., particularly among middle aged men, had increased dramatically. Biochemist Ancel

Keys of the University of Minnesota, Twin Cities, was among the first to suggest that dietary fats might be the cause. During the war, Keys had been in charge of determining the nutritional requirements of soldiers and designing portable ready-made meals. (His last name lent the "K" to K rations.) During the war, Keys studied starvation and subsistence diets, eventually producing his two-volume *Biology of Human Starvation* in 1950.[10]

After the war, Keys returned to his position as director of the Laboratory of Physiological Hygiene at the University of Minnesota, a position he held from 1939 until his retirement in 1975. His interest in diet and cardiovascular disease was prompted by data that struck him as paradoxical: American business executives, presumably among the best-fed people in the world, experienced high rates of heart disease, while in post-war Europe cardiovascular disease rates had decreased sharply in the wake of reduced food supplies. Postulating a correlation between cholesterol levels and cardiovascular disease, Keys initiated a study of Minnesota businessmen that ultimately claimed strong associations among cardiovascular disease rates, levels of serum cholesterol, and intake of saturated fatty acids.[11]

Following up on the Minnesota study, Keys and a team of scientists embarked on the "Seven Countries" study[12], which took 20 years to complete. This research compared dietary patterns to cardiovascular disease rates among 13,000 men aged 40-59 years in seven countries: Italy, Greece, Yugoslavia, the Netherlands, Finland, the United States, and Japan. The Seven Countries study claimed scientific proof that a diet low in animal products and saturated fat was associated with low mean population levels of serum cholesterol and low incidence and mortality from coronary heart disease. The scientists concluded that "population death rates from coronary heart disease can be predicted precisely by knowledge of the average serum cholesterol."

Additionally, this study claimed that intake of monounsaturated fatty acids had a strong inverse relationship with "coronary, cancer and all-cause mortality." This claim was based primarily on data from Greece, where the diet was rich in legumes, fruit, and edible fats that were mostly olive oil. The study reported that the rate of premature death from heart attack was 90 percent lower for Greek men than for American men. (Greece had 48 deaths per 100,000 population from ischemic heart disease in men aged 50-54, while the United States had 466.) Additionally, rates of other chronic diseases were also found to be low throughout Greece (the prevalence of breast cancer, for example, was one-fourth that of Japan), and the life expectancy of Greek male adults was the highest in the world. Further, rates of most chronic diseases now thought to be diet-related were lower in Greece than anywhere else.

In essence, the Seven Countries study provided compelling evidence that high intake of saturated fat increases cardiovascular disease and other poor health outcomes, while high intake of unsaturated fat decreases cardiovascular disease and other poor health outcomes. For some reason, however, the distinction between the adverse effects of saturated fat and the beneficial effects of monounsaturated fat seems to have been missed or ignored by the American medical and nutritional establishment, which ultimately concluded that *all* dietary fat is unhealthy, and launched the low-fat movement in America.

This effort blossomed in the early 1960s when the Framingham Heart Study linked cholesterol levels to heart disease[13] and the American Heart

> *Following the low-fat diet may be an early example of "political correctness."*

Association began advocating a diet low in all fats. Throughout the 1960s the low-fat movement flourished, fueled in part by the countercultural bent for revamping every facet of American society. In retrospect, the eagerness to follow the antiestablishment low-fat diet may be an early example of what has since been termed "political correctness."

By the end of the decade, a prominent group of scientists had become concerned that the low-fat diet might actually have detrimental health consequences. The 1969 Diet-Heart Review Panel of the National

Heart Institute (now the National Heart, Lung, and Blood Institute) was comprised of ten experts in clinical medicine, epidemiology, human nutrition, metabolism and biostatistics, who expressed concern that a low-fat diet could adversely affect brain chemistry, cellular aging, and the clotting ability of blood cells. These scientists knew that the only way to accurately determine the effects of a low-fat diet on the human body would be to conduct a large-scale longitudinal study involving thousands of people. The health of Americans who switched to low-fat diets could be compared over many years to an equal number of people who maintained the fat content of their existing diets. Unwilling to commit the estimated $1 billion and 10 years required to complete such a study, the National Institutes of Health embarked on a series of smaller trials beginning in the early 1970s.

When in Doubt, Ignore the Data

The scientific studies intended to bear out the emerging "fat is bad" philosophy not only failed to prove that reduced consumption of fat would yield beneficial health consequences, but generally demonstrated just the opposite. One of these studies compared disease rates and diet among men in the cities of Honolulu, Puerto Rico, Chicago, and Framingham, but failed to produce any evidence that men who consumed less fat lived longer or had fewer heart attacks.[14-16] Another study, the Multiple Risk Factor Intervention Trial, demonstrated that eating less fat might actually *shorten* lifespan. Faced with evidence that disproved their biases, the researchers discounted the results, attributing the dissatisfying results to methodological flaws.[17]

> *The scientific studies intended to bear out the "fat is bad" philosophy generally demonstrated just the opposite.*

In 1980, Philip Handler, president of the National Academy of Sciences, testified in Congress, pleading for a reconsideration of the low-fat diet recommendation. "What right," he asked, "has the federal government to propose that the American people conduct a vast nutritional experiment, with themselves as subjects, on the strength of so very little evidence that it will do them any good?"[18] Handler's plea, however, failed to derail the low-fat juggernaut.

Despite the lack of conclusive evidence that the low-fat diet produced health benefits, the U.S. Senate Select Committee on Nutrition and Human Needs issued a report in 1977 entitled *Dietary Goals for the United States,*[19] that claimed all Americans ages two and older should:

1. Increase carbohydrate consumption to 55-60 percent of caloric intake.

2. Reduce overall fat consumption to 30 percent of caloric intake.

While many Americans undoubtedly assume that these dietary goals were based on empirical evidence of their efficacy, a review of the process that led to the report's publication reveals that they were created not by scientists, but by politicians and journalists.

Science writer Gary Taubes claims "it was Senator George McGovern's bipartisan, non-legislative Select Committee on Nutrition and Human Needs–and, to be precise, a handful of McGovern's staff members–that almost single-handedly changed nutritional policy in this country and initiated the process of turning the dietary fat hypothesis into dogma."[18] The McGovern committee was established in 1968 and charged with the eradication not of overweight but of malnutrition in America. According to Taubes, when the committee's work on malnutrition was completed in the mid-1970s, two young lawyers on the committee–general counsel Marshall Matz and staff director Alan Stone–decided that instead of disbanding, the committee should change its focus from malnutrition to overconsumption. Matz later admitted, "We really were totally naïve, a bunch of kids, who just thought, 'Hell, we should say something on this subject before we go out of business.'"[18]

In July 1976, McGovern's committee listened to two days of testimony on diet and disease, then assigned the task of researching and writing the report to Nick Mottern, a former labor reporter for *The Providence Journal*. According to Taubes, "Mottern saw dietary fat as the nutritional equivalent of cigarettes, and the food industry as akin to the tobacco industry in its willingness to suppress scientific truth in the interests of profits." Although he apparently had no experience or expertise in science, nutrition, or health, Mottern was convinced his report would launch a "revolution in diet and agriculture."

The "Dietary Goals for the United States" appear to have been based not on scientific evidence but on idealism and conjecture.

Consequently, Mottern's report, entitled "Dietary Goals for the United States," recommended a significant increase in the consumption of carbohydrates and a severe reduction of dietary fat. While the report acknowledged the existence of controversy, it insisted there was nothing to lose by following this diet. "The question to be asked is not why should we change our diet but why not?" wrote Harvard School of Public Health nutritionist Mark Hegsted in the introduction. "There are [no risks] that can be identified and important benefits can be expected."

Based on Taubes' analysis of the the McGovern committee proceedings, the recommendations of which have formed the foundation of the U.S. Government's approach to national nutrition for the last quarter century, the "Dietary Goals for the United States" appear to have been based not on scientific evidence but on idealism and conjecture.

49

The Food Guide Pyramid

Since the publication of the 1977 McGovern committee report, no effort to codify the low-fat dogma has been as successful and far-reaching as the USDA Food Guide Pyramid. In 1988, the USDA began to develop a graphic presentation of the food guide which ultimately led to the publication of the Food Guide Pyramid in 1992. (Figure 4)

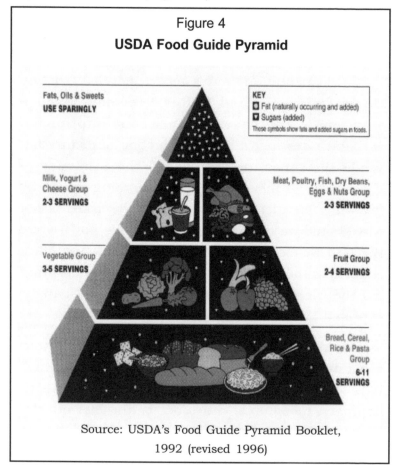

Figure 4
USDA Food Guide Pyramid

Fats, Oils & Sweets
USE SPARINGLY

KEY
☐ Fat (naturally occurring and added)
◆ Sugars (added)
These symbols show fats and added sugars in foods.

Milk, Yogurt & Cheese Group
2-3 SERVINGS

Meat, Poultry, Fish, Dry Beans, Eggs & Nuts Group
2-3 SERVINGS

Vegetable Group
3-5 SERVINGS

Fruit Group
2-4 SERVINGS

Bread, Cereal, Rice & Pasta Group
6-11 SERVINGS

Source: USDA's Food Guide Pyramid Booklet, 1992 (revised 1996)

From a broad base of six to 11 servings of bread, cereal, rice, and pasta, the pyramid narrows upward to fewer servings of vegetables and fruits, to fewer still of dairy products and meat. Finally, at the top of the pyramid are fats, oils, and sweets, which consumers are advised to "eat sparingly." In short, the pyramid recommends heavy consumption of carbohydrates and severely limited intake of fat.

> *A diet based on the Food Guide Pyramid is not only unlikely to produce weight loss, but virtually guarantees weight gain.*

When the Food Guide Pyramid was initially published, millions of Americans accepted its recommendations as the gospel truth and began fastidiously avoiding fat while consuming higher quantities of carbohydrates. In his bestselling 1995 book entitled *Enter the Zone*,[20] Barry Sears, Ph.D. referred to this as "the great carbohydrate experiment." Sears and others claim this "experiment" not only failed to help Americans lose weight, but actually made them fatter. Another obesity researcher, David Ludwig, M.D., Ph.D., at Children's Hospital in Boston, asserts that people are getting fat not because they eat too much fat but because they eat too many refined carbohydrates, which he says "may increase risk for obesity, Type-2 diabetes, and heart disease."[21] For this reason, many experts believe a diet based on the Food Guide Pyramid is not only unlikely to produce weight loss, but virtually guarantees weight gain.

Summary

Adherence to the dietary guidelines of the Food Guide Pyramid appears to have significantly contributed to the epidemic of overweight and obesity in the United States. Based on these recommendations, Americans radically altered their diets expecting to lose weight but instead gaining weight and experiencing a host of related health problems. In short, it seems to be no coincidence that the number of overweight Americans has risen 61 percent since the Food Guide Pyramid was introduced. In retrospect, the government appears to have developed and promoted dietary guidelines which have exacerbated the very problems they were intended to solve.

Cause 5. Restaurants

Meals Away From Home

Americans are eating an unprecedented percentage of meals away from home. As shown in Table 5, from 1977 to 1995 the percentage of meals eaten away from home nearly doubled (from 16 percent to 29 percent[22]), an increase that closely parallels the rise in obesity during the same time period. By 1995, one third of meals eaten away from home–or nearly one out of every 10 total meals consumed–were purchased at fast food restaurants. Thus, by the mid

1990s, Americans were eating an average of 23 meals per month away from home, with eight of those meals being consumed at fast food restaurants.

	1977-78	1987-88	1989	1990	1991	1994	1995
Table 5							
Meal and snack eating patterns of Americans							
				Number			
Meals per day	2.7	2.6	2.6	2.6	2.6	2.7	2.6
Snacks per day	1.1	0.9	1.2	1.2	1.4	1.5	1.6
				Percent			
Meals away from home	16	24	24	23	27	28	29
Snacks away from home	17	20	20	18	18	21	22
				Percent			
All meals and snacks away from home	16	23	23	22	24	26	27
Restaurant	2	4	4	4	4	6	5
Fast food	3	7	7	7	7	8	9
School*	3	2	2	2	3	2	2
Other public	3	2	2	2	2	2	2
Others	6	8	8	7	8	8	9

* Classified as a separate category for children only; for adults, they are included in "others."

Source: USDA Economic Research Service

The increased frequency of dining out has resulted in Americans consuming more of their nutrients away from home. Table 6 shows that in the late 1970s foods eaten away from home comprised 18 percent of total calories consumed. By the end of the next decade, this figure had jumped to 27 percent. By 1995, Americans were ingesting more than a third (34%) of total calories away from home. A USDA survey revealed that by 1995 school-age children were getting more than 40 percent of calories away from home.[23]

	1977-78	1987-88	1989	1990	1991	1994	1995
Calories	18	27	27	26	29	31	34
Total fat	18	28	29	28	32	35	38
Saturated fat	NA	28	29	28	31	33	37
Cholesterol	NA	26	25	25	30	32	34
Sodium	NA	27	26	26	30	32	34
Fiber	NA	22	23	22	25	26	27
Calcium	17	23	23	22	25	26	29
Iron	16	22	22	21	25	26	27

Table 6

Consumption of selected nutrients and food components in away-from-home foods,[1] as part of total diet, 1977-95

Percent of Total Diet

NA = Not available.

[1]Includes fast food restaurants, other restaurants, schools, and other public places.

Source: USDA Economic Research Service

In 1997, more than 71 percent of families in the U.S. purchased meals at restaurants, carry-outs, and other eating establishments during an average week. This represented an average annual expenditure of $1,477 per family, or nearly 31 percent of total expenditures for food.[24] Since this data was collected, our lives have become busier and busier, so there is reason to believe that the trend to consume more meals away from home has continued to increase. Though some would suggest that the solution to

The problem seems to have less to do with where we eat than what we eat.

the epidemic of overweight is to stop eating so many meals away from home, the problem appears to have less to do with *where* we eat than *what* we eat.

Fast Food Frenzy

In its early days, fast food was a treat. Because it was consumed infrequently, not much attention was given to its nutritional value. After all, we were splurging. Overeating was simply a part (if not the point) of the experience. Over the years, fast food has evolved from an occasional treat to a staple of the American diet. Fast food consumption has become so ingrained in our lifestyle that, according to the U.S. Department of Agriculture, the average American now consumes 28 pounds of French fries per year.[25] Although the frequency of fast food consumption has changed, our "splurge mentality" has not. Thus, we continue to overeat at practically every visit, which now occurs an average of eight times per month.

A review of the nutritional information provided by fast food restaurants reveals the extent of our gluttony. Take for example the McDonald's Quarter Pounder® with Cheese meal, which consists of a quarter-pound hamburger with cheese, a large serving of French fries, and a 16-ounce drink. If a sugar-free drink is selected, this meal contains 1,080 calories. With a sugar-sweetened drink, the calorie total increases to 1,230, which is 62 percent of the recommended daily intake on a 2,000 calorie diet. At

Burger King, the Whopper® with Cheese meal contains 1,300 calories with a diet drink and 1,450 calories with a sugar-sweetened drink (72% of recommended daily intake).

"Super Size" It

The problem of fast food gluttony has been intensified by a phenomenon called "upsizing" (also knows as "super sizing" or "biggie sizing"). This practice started when fast food marketers discovered they could increase profits by selling larger portions of French fries and soft drinks. The downside of upsizing is that it can increase the total calories of a meal by 200 calories or more. As a result, it is common to consume more than 80 percent of the recommended number of daily calories in one fast food meal.

> *It is common to consume more than 80 percent of the recommended number of daily calories in one fast food meal.*

In light of the caloric excess of many fast food offerings, it is easy to see why this industry is often blamed for the epidemic of obesity, as evidenced by a number of lawsuits filed against McDonald's by people who blame the company for their obesity and weight-related health problems. In his book, *Fast Food Nation: The Dark Side of the All-American Meal*[26], author Eric Schlosser blames much of the increase in childhood obesity on the fast-food industry. Schlosser is particularly offended by the way the fast food giants have focused advertising and marketing on children, and recommends that Congress enact laws to ban fast-food advertising aimed at children under the age of nine.

The Unhappy Meal

For children in America, fast food has become a regular dietary component. In one of the first studies to examine the effects of fast food consumption on childhood nutrition and health-related outcomes, Dr. David Ludwig, director of the obesity program at Children's Hospital Boston, led a team of researchers who examined the diets of 6,212 U.S. children and adolescents from1994 to 1998, and found that[27]:

- On a typical day, more than 30 percent of 4-19 year-olds consumed fast food.

- Fast-food consumption was highly prevalent in both genders, all racial/ethnic groups, and all regions of the country.

- Those who ate fast food consumed more:
    - Total energy (187 kilocalories)
    - Energy per gram of food (0.29 kcal/g)
    - Total carbohydrates (24 g)
    - Added sugars (26 g)
    - Sugar-sweetened beverages (228 g)

- Children who ate fast food consumed less fiber (-1.1 g) and milk (-65 g), as well as fruits and nonstarchy vegetables (-45 g).

- Eating fast food increased a child's weight an average of six extra pounds per year.

Very important ✳

While there is no doubt that fast food has contributed significantly to the epidemic of childhood overweight and obesity, those who place all of the blame on the fast food industry seem to ignore two important facts:

FACT #1: Young children do not drive cars or earn income. Therefore:

FACT #2: Someone must be taking children to fast food restaurants and paying for their food.

Overwhelmingly, it is parents, grandparents, and other adults who not only provide the transportation and funding, but also place the orders. Imagine if the prize in every kid's meal were a pack of cigarettes and a book of matches. Would we still order our children so many fast food meals? Yet the health risks associated with heavy consumption of hamburgers, French fries, and soft drinks appear to be as severe as the risks of smoking.

> *Imagine if the prize in every kid's meal were a pack of cigarettes and a book of matches.*

An Evil Empire?

There are those who seem to believe that the executives at McDonald's, Burger King, Wendy's, and other fast food chains have concocted an evil scheme to murder us with their delicious but deadly fare. Such conspiracy theories, however, do not bear scrutiny. In the highly competitive business climate in which they operate, fast food companies probably do not have the time or resources to plot the demise of humanity. Instead, the ultimate aim of these companies, like every other business enterprise, is to maximize revenue and profit. Doing so benefits employees, stockholders, and ultimately the national economy. Consequently, attempting to put fast food companies out of business seems un-American.

> **Fast food companies would prefer to generate revenue and profit with products that promote health rather than diminish it.**

Healthy Fast Food

In all likelihood, fast food companies would prefer to generate revenue and profit with products that promote health rather than diminish it. They know that customers want more nutritious fare, and several have attempted to provide it. According to the National Restaurant Association:

"To cater to increasingly health-conscious diners, restaurants across the country are increasing their efforts to provide what their guests ask for, including developing special menu items for those watching their calorie and/or fat intake, voluntarily providing nutritional information in brochures and on Web sites, and establishing their own initiatives to assist consumers live a healthy lifestyle."[28]

Despite these efforts, most attempts by fast food restaurants to sell healthier food have not been successful. One reason is the apparent disconnect between what consumers say they want and what they actually purchase. Although surveys have consistently shown that patrons claim to want more nutritious menu items, when these items are actually offered they generally do not sell well because customers continue to order the standard fare (hamburgers, French fries, etc.). Another reason is that fast food restaurants have tended to focus on reducing fat rather than carbohydrates. Consequently, many of their "healthy" alternatives are not much more nutritious than traditional menu items, and, because they still contain

> *A number of fast food companies have responded to requests for low-carbohydrate, rather than low-fat, items.*

high levels of carbohydrates and sugar, some are more fattening than the traditional menu items. Recently, several fast food companies have responded to customer requests for low-carbohydrate, rather than low-fat, items. Only time will tell if customers are willing to put their money where their mouths are by purchasing these lower-carbohydrate offerings, or whether the restaurants can profitably deliver them.

Traditional Restaurants

Several table service restaurants have also publicized efforts to provide more healthful menu items. However, like the fast food companies, many have made the mistake of focusing on fat rather than carbohydrates. Additionally, at many table service restaurants, the worst concentration of fattening foods is found on the Children's Menu. At most restaurants, the Children's Menu typically contains any or all of the following items:

- Grilled cheese sandwich

- Pizza

- Macaroni and cheese

- Spaghetti

- Hamburger and French fries

- Chicken fingers and French fries

- Hot dog and French fries

Chapter Four will explain why these items are so unhealthy, and Chapter Five will present a strategy for feeding children nutritious meals in restaurants. For now, suffice it to say that

> **Allowing children to order from the Children's Menu virtually guarantees an unhealthy meal.**

allowing children to order from the Children's Menu virtually guarantees an unhealthy meal.

Cause 6. Schools

The National School Lunch Program

Each school day, more than 26 million children get their lunches through the USDA's National School Lunch Program (NSLP). This program was established in 1946 by the National School Lunch Act which mandated that school meals "safeguard the health and well-being of the Nation's children."[29] Today, this federally assisted meal program provides low-cost or free lunches in more than 99,800 schools and child care institutions. The cost of the program has grown from $70 million in 1947 to 6.4 billion in FY 2001.[29]

Institutions that qualify for the program are public or nonprofit private schools and public or nonprofit private residential child care facilities. For each meal they serve, school districts and independent schools that choose to take part in the program receive cash subsidies and donated commodities from the U.S. Department of Agriculture. In return, they must serve lunches that meet federal requirements, and they must offer free or reduced price lunches to eligible children. Reimbursement is also offered for snacks served in after-school educational and enrichment programs.

Between 1994 and 1996 about half of all students attending schools that offered the NSLP ate a school lunch on any given day.[29] Among participating students, 36 percent received free meals, 8 percent received reduced-price meals, and the remainder paid the full price.[30] In terms of nutritional content, school lunches have only two requirements:[29]

1. Must provide no more than 30 percent of calories from fat, and less than 10 percent from saturated fat.

2. Must provide at least one third of the Recommended Dietary Allowance (RDA) of calories, protein, Vitamin A, Vitamin C, iron, and calcium.

Decisions about what specific foods to serve and how they are prepared are made by local school food authorities.[29]

Most of the support the USDA provides to schools in the NSLP comes in the form of a cash reimbursement for each meal served. In addition to cash reimbursements, schools are entitled by law to receive commodity foods, called "entitlement" foods, at a value of 15.75 cents for each meal served. Schools can also get "bonus" commodities as they are made available from

The school lunch program not only feeds children, but also creates a market for unwanted food commodities, a practice that can conflict with the mandate to "safeguard the health and well-being of the nation's children."

surplus agricultural stocks. Thus, the school lunch program not only feeds children, but also creates a market for unwanted food commodities, a practice that can conflict with the mandate to "safeguard the health and well-being of the nation's children."

The current basic cash reimbursement rates for the NSLP are shown in Table 7.

Table 7		
USDA National School Lunch Program		
Reimbursement Rates: July 1, 2004 through June 30, 2005		
	Free	Reduced-Price	Paid
Lunch	$2.24	$1.84	$0.21
Snacks	$0.61	$0.30	$0.05

Because they struggle to break even on these federal subsidies, many schools have found other ways to increase revenue from food and beverages.

Press "A-8" for Overweight

The majority of the nation's schools now contain vending machines. According to a study of school health policies and programs by the Centers for Disease Control and Prevention, vending machines are present in 43 percent of elementary schools, 74 percent of middle schools, and nearly every high school. Although it is the official policy of the National School Lunch Program that vending machines are not to operate in cafeterias during lunch hours, the CDC study revealed that most schools disobey this rule, as vending machines were operated during lunch hours in 68 percent of schools that had them.[31]

> *Vending machines are in 43% of elementary schools, 74% of middle schools, and nearly every high school.*

Because they typically contain high-calorie, high-carbohydrate foods such as chips, crackers, cookies, and candy, it is virtually impossible to find a nutritious snack in a vending machine. By washing down one of these snacks with a sugar-sweetened soft drink, it is common for children to consume 500-1,000 empty calories between classes, a practice some children repeat several times per day.

To further increase revenue from soft drinks, many school districts have accepted "exclusive pouring rights" contracts in which soft drink manufacturers pay the school to promote their brand exclusively.[32]

Bonus incentives are frequently included in these contracts to encourage schools to promote sales.[33] Thus, these contracts can put schools in the position of encouraging students to consume fattening

> **Many school districts have contracts in which soft drink manufacturers pay the school to promote their brand exclusively.**

beverages. Nonetheless, many school officials seem to disregard the health risks these contracts pose to students, claiming that the financial gains benefit students, schools, communities, and taxpayers.[34]

From the Lunch Line to the Waistline

In addition to the money they make from vending machines, 56 percent of schools generate additional revenue by offering premium-priced entrees such as pizza, hamburgers, and sandwiches.[35] While many of these items would violate the nutritional requirements of the National School Lunch Program, because they are sold a la carte, these items are exempt from the dietary guidelines of the NSLP.[29] This phenomenon seems to present a conflict of interest in which the school derives the greatest financial benefit when students select the least nutritious foods.

Reading, Writing, and Fast Food

Another source of additional revenue for schools is generated by allowing fast food companies to offer their fare on campus. According to the Centers for Disease Control, 20 percent of public schools now offer brand-name fast food as an alternative to cafeteria meals. This is a dramatic increase from 1991, when only two percent of

> *20 percent of public schools now offer brand-name fast food as an alternative to cafeteria meals.*

public schools participating in the National School Lunch Program sold brand-name fast foods. The state of California, which prides itself on being a national trendsetter, appears to be leading the country on this measure as well. In a survey conducted in February of 2000, 53 percent of responding California school districts reported that their high schools offered food from Taco Bell, 22 percent from Subway, and 19 percent from Domino's.[36]

One of the popular fast foods offered in schools is the Pizza Hut Personal Pan Pizza. According to Pizza Hut's nutrition information[37], a Supreme Personal Pan Pizza contains 760 calories, 72 grams of carbohydrates and 1,680 mg. of sodium (72 percent of the Recommended Dietary Allowance). In its nutritional data sheet, the company elegantly hides this information by reporting a serving size of only one slice, or one quarter of the contents of the box (Table 8). Consuming this pizza with a 12-ounce sugar-sweetened soft drink adds another 150 to 200 calories, 40 carbohydrates, and 40 grams of sugar, bringing the total lunch consumption (assuming no dessert) to over 900 calories and 110 grams of carbohydrates.

Table 8					
Pizza Hut 6″ Personal Pan Pizza Nutrition Data					
6″ Personal Pan Pizza®	**Serving Size**	**Calories**	**Carbohy-drates (g)**	**Sodium (mg)**	**% Daily Value**
Cheese	Slice	160	18	310	13
Pepperoni	Slice	170	18	340	14
Quartered Ham	Slice	150	18	330	14
Supreme	Slice	190	19	420	18
Super Supreme	Slice	200	19	480	20
Chicken Supreme	Slice	160	19	320	13
Meat Lover's	Slice	200	18	470	20
Veggie Lover's	Slice	150	19	280	12
Pepperoni Lover's	Slice	200	18	440	18
Sausage Lover's	Slice	190	18	400	70
Source: Pizza Hut Website					

Some school systems have foregone these contracts and banned the sale of soft drinks and fast food in their schools. In California, for example, the Los Angeles Unified School District decided to ban soft drinks in all schools, and the California state legislature passed a law banning or limiting sales in elementary and middle schools. Similarly, Texas commissioner of agriculture Susan Combs issued a ban on consumption of soft drinks and other non-nutritious foods in Texas elementary schools.

Actions like these have frightened soft drink manufacturers and fast food chains into becoming more vocal advocates of nutrition and exercise. For example, in an effort to keep the focus on *increasing* physical activity rather than *decreasing* soft drink consumption, the Coca-Cola Company has publicized its official position that "rising obesity rates are due in large part to sedentary lifestyles and lack of physical activity," and that "soft drinks can be part of an active lifestyle."[38] Coke has also partnered with the National Association for Sport and Physical Education (NASPE) to offer the "Step With It" exercise program in schools across the country. This program provides children a device to measure the number of steps they take, and encourages them to accumulate a total of 10,000 steps per day. PepsiCo has taken a position similar to its rival, claiming "Sixty percent of the increase in obesity in the U.S. is most likely due to less physical activity brought on by things like computers and too much television. A recent National Bureau of Economic Research study found that physical activity at home and at work decreased significantly between 1976 and 1994."[39]

To inform pediatricians, other health care professionals, parents, superintendents, and school board members about nutritional concerns regarding soft drink consumption in schools, the American Academy of Pediatrics (AAP) issued a policy statement in January 2004 called "Soft Drinks in Schools."[40] This policy recommended that:

- Pediatricians advocate for the creation of a school nutrition advisory council as one means of ensuring that the health and nutritional interests of students form the foundation of nutritional policies in schools.

- School districts should invite public discussion before making any decision to sign a vended food or drink contract.

- If a school district already has a soft drink contract in place, it should be adapted so that it does not promote overconsumption by students.

- Consumption or advertising of sweetened soft drinks within the classroom should be eliminated.

- Vending machines should not be placed within the cafeteria space where lunch is sold.

- Soft drinks should not be sold as part of, or in competition with, the school lunch program.

Summary

The problem with the food being served to our nation's schoolchildren appears to be caused by two conflicts of interest. The first is found in the National School Lunch Program which, at a cost of $6.4 billion dollars per year, seeks to fulfill the seemingly incompatible objectives of providing nutritious meals to schoolchildren while simultaneously creating a dumping ground for unwanted food products. The second conflict of interest pits the obligation of each school to provide nutritious meals against the revenue which can be generated by selling fast food and soft drinks. In the

> *Many schools need to do a better job of providing nutritious meals and snacks to students.*

final analysis, it appears that many schools need to do a better job of providing nutritious meals and snacks to students.

Cause 7. Lack of Exercise

Compounding the problem of poor nutrition in schools is a drastic reduction in physical education. P.E. was once an important part of every child's school day. Today only 8 percent of elementary schools, 6.4 percent of middle/junior high schools, and 5.8 percent of senior high schools provide daily physical education or its equivalent (150 minutes per week for elementary schools; 225 minutes per week for middle/junior and senior high schools) for the entire school year for students in all grades in the school.[41] Although virtually all parents, educators, and health professionals acknowledge the merits of quality, daily physical education, Illinois is currently the only state that requires daily physical education for students in kindergarten through 12th grade.

Outside of the classroom, there is an equally severe lack of physical activity. For example, among children ages 9-13, one fifth of boys and one fourth of girls engage in no free-time physical activity.[42] Among high school students (grades 9-12):[43]

- 31% do not achieve recommended levels of physical activity (Figure 5).

- 48% are not enrolled in a physical education class. Enrollment drops from 74% for ninth graders to 31% for 12th graders.

- Daily participation in high school physical education classes decreased from 42% in 1991 to 32% in 2001.

- Girls are much less likely than boys to engage in regular vigorous physical activity.

- African-American and Hispanic youth tend to be less vigorously active than white youth.

- Participation in physical activity decreases as grade level increases. Regular participation in vigorous-intensity physical activity drops from 72% for ninth graders to 56% for 12th graders.

- 45% do not play on sports teams during the year.

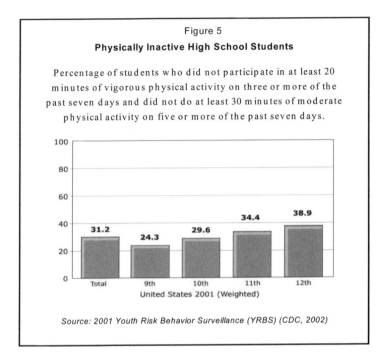

Figure 5

Physically Inactive High School Students

Percentage of students who did not participate in at least 20 minutes of vigorous physical activity on three or more of the past seven days and did not do at least 30 minutes of moderate physical activity on five or more of the past seven days.

United States 2001 (Weighted)

Source: 2001 Youth Risk Behavior Surveillance (YRBS) (CDC, 2002)

While the federal government recommends that children and adolescents accumulate at least 60 minutes of moderate physical activity most days of the week,[44] few young people achieve this level of activity. With 20 percent of U.S. children participating in two or fewer vigorous physical activities per week[45], it is clear that many children have adopted sedentary lifestyles.

Many children have adopted sedentary lifestyles.

73

Cause 8. Sugar

Most parents know that sugar causes tooth decay, but few realize the extent to which sugar has contributed to the epidemic of overweight and Type 2 diabetes. In the last 40 years, sugar consumption in America has increased at an extraordinary rate.

> *Most parents know that sugar causes tooth decay, but few realize the extent to which sugar has contributed to the epidemic of overweight and Type 2 diabetes.*

According to the USDA, average annual consumption of caloric sweeteners in the United States increased by 22 percent between 1980 and 2000.[46] By the mid 1990s, school-age children in America were consuming 20 percent of total daily calories in the form of added sugars.[47]

As shown in Figure 6, in the period 1994-1996, school-age children consumed an average of more than half a cup (26 teaspoons) of added sugar per day. Added sugar consumption ranged from 19 teaspoons per day for 6-8 year-old girls to 36 teaspoons (1.5 cups) for 14-18 year-old boys.[48]

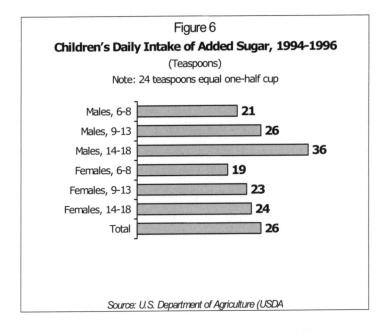

Figure 6

Children's Daily Intake of Added Sugar, 1994-1996

(Teaspoons)

Note: 24 teaspoons equal one-half cup

Category	Teaspoons
Males, 6-8	21
Males, 9-13	26
Males, 14-18	36
Females, 6-8	19
Females, 9-13	23
Females, 14-18	24
Total	26

Source: U.S. Department of Agriculture (USDA

Liquid Candy

The chief source of the increased consumption of sugar is soft drinks.[49] Between 1979 and 1996, children's soft drink consumption increased by 300 percent.[50] Average serving sizes have increased from 6.5 oz. in the 1950s to 12 oz. in the 1960s to 20 oz. by the late 1990s. Today, soft drinks are commonly purchased in portions as large as 48 ounces. An average 12-oz. carbonated, sugar-sweetened soft drink contains 41 grams (about 10 teaspoons) of sugar and 150 calories. Thus, a 48-oz. sugar-sweetened soft drink contains 600 calories and 164 grams–about 40 teaspoons-of sugar.

Between 56 percent and 85 percent of school-age children consume at least one soft drink daily, with the highest amounts ingested by adolescent males, 20 percent of whom consume four or

> *A 48-ounce sugar-sweetened soft drink contains 600 calories and 40 teaspoons of sugar.*

more servings per day.[51] Research has shown that children who consume soft drinks have a higher daily calorie intake than nonconsumers.[51] Each additional 12-oz. sugar-sweetened soft drink consumed per day has been associated with a 0.18-point increase in a child's BMI and a 60 percent increase in the risk of obesity.[52] Although sugar-free soft drinks do not carry these risks,[52] they constitute only 14 percent of the adolescent soft drink market.[53]

In addition to carbonated soft drinks, children have dramatically increased consumption of fruit-flavored drinks. The FDA mandates that beverages cannot be labeled as fruit juice unless they contain 100 percent fruit juice. Any beverage that is less than that must list the percentage of the product that is fruit juice, and the beverage must include a descriptive term such as "drink," "beverage," or "cocktail."[54] In general, juice drinks contain 10 to 99 percent juice, sweeteners such as sugar or high fructose corn syrup, flavors, and in some cases fortifiers such as vitamin C or calcium. Water is the main ingredient of fruit drinks, with carbohydrates, including sucrose, fructose, glucose, and sorbitol, being the next most prevalent component.

Historically, fruit juice was recommended by pediatricians as a source of vitamin C and an extra source of water for healthy infants and young children. The introduction of the juice box and later the juice pouch created an enormous boom for fruit drink sales by creating a product delivery system that was highly convenient and transportable. Suddenly, parents had the ability to take juice drinks wherever they took their children. Evidently that is exactly what many parents have done, based largely on the convenience factor and the erroneous assumption that fruit-flavored drinks promote health.

Overconsumption of 100 percent fruit juice also appears to be contributing to childhood overweight. A recent study conducted by Dr. Sarita Dhuper, director of pediatric cardiology and the pediatric obesity clinic at the Brookdale University Hospital and Medical Center, showed that overweight children consume 65 percent more fruit juice than thinner kids.[55] "Parents think that because fruit juices are natural that they are a healthy drink, so they don't put a limit on how much their children consume," said Dr. Dhuper. "Our study found that juice consumption is almost shocking. For some kids, there seems to be no limit to what they can drink in a given day."[56]

Another study found a link between obesity and juice intake in excess of 12 ounces per day.[57] The American Academy of Pediatrics recommends that fruit juice intake be limited to 4-6 ounces per day for children ages one to six, and 8-12 ounces a day for children ages seven to eighteen. Nevertheless, it is quite common for children to consume ten times the recommended amount every day. Although these drinks do not contain added sugars or artificial sweeteners, they still

> *Parents should wean children from soft drinks and replace these beverages with water.*

contain significant amounts of sugar, a problem that is often overlooked by parents and other adults.

The problem of overconsumption of sugar in beverages is exacerbated by two facts:

1. Consuming sugar is particularly fattening when ingested in liquid form.[58]

2. These drinks represent calories added to, rather than displacing, other dietary intake.[59, 60]

The implication is clear: parents should wean children from soft drinks and replace these beverages with water.

Pass the Syrup

Another factor in the increased consumption of sugar is the enormous rise in the use of corn sweeteners, including high fructose corn syrup (HFCS). Because HFCS has a chemical structure similar to sucrose but is much less expensive than raw sugar, it is a highly profitable ingredient for food and drink manufacturers, and is now commonly used in a variety of products including beverages, cereal and baked goods, dairy products, candy, and many other processed foods. Production of HFCS in the U.S. increased from 2.2 million tons in 1980 to 9.4

> *Much of the sugar children ingest is stored as fat.*

million tons in 1999, and now consumes more than five percent of the total U.S. corn crop.[61]

Summary

Overconsumption of sugar is a widespread problem among children. Because of the way the body metabolizes carbohydrates (see Chapter Four), much of the sugar children ingest is stored as fat. Combining a high intake of added sugar with a diet high in other carbohydrates appears to significantly increase the risk of both overweight and Type 2 diabetes.

Cause 9. Parents

It has long been observed that overweight "runs in families." In fact, research has shown that the most reliable predictor of weight problems in young children is whether or not their parents are overweight.[62] For young children with one obese parent, the odds are approximately three to one that the child will suffer obesity in adulthood. If both parents are obese, the odds are more than ten to one. Parental obesity is such a strong predictor that by the time a child reaches age three, parental weight is a stronger predictor of the child's future weight than the child's own weight.[63]

Based on such evidence, one might conclude that the problem of childhood overweight is genetic. However, while some scientists believe that heredity can cause a predisposition to overweight, unless there has been a significant change in the genetic makeup of Americans in the last 25 years, heredity simply cannot account for the dramatic rise in the prevalence of overweight children. Thus, environment and behavior must have a greater impact on weight than genetics. Because the child's environment and behavior are both shaped predominantly by parents, ultimately it appears that the most significant way

> **The most significant way parents contribute to the problem of childhood overweight is by creating or tolerating the environment and behaviors that promote it.**

parents contribute to the problem of childhood overweight is by creating or tolerating the environment and behaviors that promote it.

For example, most parents know that children need more exercise, yet many allow their children to spend hours each day on passive activities such as television, video games, and the Internet. Most parents also know that children need to eat healthful foods, yet many provide or allow their children a steady diet of junk food, fast food, and convenience food. Perhaps most convicting of all is the fact that parents generally understand the need to set a proper example for children, yet most continue to eat poorly and exercise too little. As a result, two out of three

> *Many parents fail to set a proper example for children with their own diet and exercise practices.*

American adults are overweight, and about half of these are obese. Thus, many parents are failing at what experts consider among the most important responsibilities of a parent: To provide for the safety and wellbeing of their children, and to model acceptable behavior.

Cause 10. Coincidence

It has been called the meteorological event of the century. In October of 1991, a storm devastated the Atlantic coast, causing a hurricane as far north as Nova Scotia, flooding as far south as the Dominican Republic, and the deaths of six fishermen aboard the *Andrea Gail* off the coast of Gloucester, Massachusetts. The subject of a bestselling book and subsequent movie, this tempest was created by a rare combination of factors that resulted in a storm stronger than any in recorded history.

When it began, this storm was not particularly remarkable—just a typical "nor'easter." What caused it to become "The Perfect Storm" was a rare combination of forces: As the Great Lakes storm moved east, a Canadian cold front moved south, and Hurricane Grace took a bizarre north turn from the Bahamas. When these three storms collided in the North Atlantic, meteorologists at the U.S. National Weather Service issued maritime warnings, but by the time they realized how truly devastating the weather had become, it was too late for Captain Billy Tynes and the crew of the Andrea Gail. Their ship was sunk by waves of 100 feet and winds in excess of 120 miles per hour.

The current epidemic of overweight children is not unlike "The Perfect Storm" —a convergence of forces in which the whole is greater than the sum of its parts. The forces that have converged on our young people include changes in society, innovation in food and technology, overconsumption of electronic media, poor nutritional advice from the government, increased consumption of high-calorie food from restaurants and fast food establishments, poor nutritional offerings and lack of exercise in schools, lack of exercise at home, increased consumption of sugar in both food and drinks, and parents who fail to set or model proper standards of nutrition and exercise. Individually, each of these factors is capable of doing considerable harm. Combined, they have wreaked havoc beyond anyone's ability to predict. The question is whether it is too late for those in the path of this storm. Are our children, like those aboard the *Andrea Gail*, ultimately doomed?

3

CONSEQUENCES

"If obesity is left unchecked, almost
all Americans will be overweight by
2050. Obesity is a normal response
to the American environment."

*– University of Colorado
physiologist James O. Hill*

Part 1. Physical Consequences

Being overweight can kill you. Each year in the United
States, approximately 300,000 deaths are associated
with overweight and obesity[1], making obesity the
second leading cause of preventable death behind
smoking. While most obesity-related deaths occur
among adults, the consequences of excess weight are
also suffered by children and adolescents. According
to the American Academy of Pediatrics, "Obesity is
associated with significant health problems in the

pediatric age group and is an important early risk factor for much of adult morbidity and mortality."[2]

> *Among overweight 5-10 year-olds, 60% already have at least one cardiovascular disease risk factor.*

Medical problems are common in obese children and adolescents. The most common complications affect the cardiovascular system (including high blood pressure, high cholesterol, and high triglycerides)[3-6] and the endocrine system (including hyperinsulinism, insulin resistance, impaired glucose tolerance, Type 2 diabetes, and menstrual irregularity).[7-9] Research has shown that among overweight 5-10 year-olds, 60 percent already have at least one cardiovascular disease risk factor.[10] Other medical problems associated with pediatric overweight and obesity include pulmonary complications (including asthma and obstructive sleep apnea syndrome),[11-16] orthopedic complications,[17, 18] and gastrointestinal/liver problems.[19]

Type 2 Diabetes

One of the more shocking medical problems associated with the epidemic of childhood overweight and obesity is the alarming increase in the incidence of Type 2 diabetes, a chronic disease that develops when the pancreas cannot produce enough insulin or when the body's tissues become resistant to insulin. When insulin is not available or is not used properly, the blood sugar level rises above what is safe. If blood sugar levels remain high for years, blood vessels and nerves throughout the body may be damaged and the risk is increased for eye, heart, blood vessel, nerve, and kidney disease. Unlike Type 1 diabetes, blood sugar levels among Type 2 diabetics rise so slowly that a person usually does not have symptoms and may have the disease for many years before diagnosis.

One of the more shocking medical problems associated with the epidemic of childhood overweight is the alarming increase in Type 2 diabetes.

Once known as "adult-onset diabetes," this disease is now so prevalent in children and adolescents that its name had to be changed. The increase of obesity in children and adolescents is reported to be the most significant factor for the rise in diabetes. Before 1992, Type 2 diabetes accounted for only 2-4 percent of all childhood diabetes. By 1994, this number had skyrocketed to 16 percent.[20] Additionally, obese children and adolescents are reported to be 12.6 times more likely to have high fasting blood insulin levels, a risk factor for Type 2 diabetes.[21] Children of certain ethnic groups are at especially high risk, with Type 2 diabetes predominating among children and adolescents of Mexican, African American, and Hispanic descent.[21]

Metabolic Syndrome

At least four percent of U.S. adolescents and 30 percent of obese adolescents are affected by metabolic syndrome, a cluster of cardiac risk factors that leads to the early onset of diabetes and heart disease.[22] Also referred to as "insulin resistance syndrome" and "syndrome X," metabolic syndrome is characterized by a combination of high blood pressure, high triglycerides, low HDL-cholesterol, high blood sugar, and abdominal obesity. The underlying causes are overweight/obesity, physical inactivity and genetic factors.[23]

Additional Complications

Research has shown that the medical complications of childhood overweight and obesity are likely to continue into adulthood,[24, 25] and the risk of obesity persisting into adulthood is higher for adolescents than for younger children.[26] The probability that childhood obesity will persist into adulthood increases from approximately 20 percent at age four to approximately 80 percent by adolescence.[27] As overweight children and adolescents become overweight adults, they experience a significantly increased risk for premature death[28] as well as a number of debilitating conditions including:[29]

- Angina pectoris

- Bladder control problems (such as stress incontinence)

- Cancer (especially endometrial, breast, prostate, and colon)

- Complications of pregnancy

- Congestive heart failure

- Coronary heart disease

- Gallstones

- Gout

- High cholesterol

- Hypertension

- Hyperinsulinemia

- Insulin resistance/Glucose intolerance

- Obstructive sleep apnea and respiratory problems

- Osteoarthritis

- Poor female reproductive health (such as menstrual irregularities, infertility, irregular ovulation)

- Psychological disorders (such as depression, eating disorders, distorted body image, and low self esteem).

- Stroke

- Type 2 (non-insulin dependent) diabetes

Part 2. Economic Consequences

ഇന്ന

"Obesity has become a crucial
health problem for our nation...
The medical costs alone reflect the
significance of the challenge."

— *Tommy Thompson, U.S. Secretary
of Health & Human Services*

ഇന്ന

The potential health care costs associated with pediatric obesity and its related complications are staggering. For the U.S. healthcare system, overweight and obesity have already created a substantial economic burden.[30, 31] Nationally, the estimated annual cost attributable to obesity-related diseases is about $100 billion.[32] About half of these costs are financed by taxpayers through Medicare and Medicaid.[33] (Medicare is a federal program for seniors and the disabled, and Medicaid is a federal and state program for the poor.) The Centers for Disease Control revealed that in 2003, 6.8 percent of total Medicare expenditures and 10.6 percent of total Medicaid expenditures were for the treatment of obesity.[33]

> *The potential health care costs associated with pediatric obesity and its related complications are staggering.*

The most frequently cited estimates of the economic costs of overweight and obesity were published in *Obesity Research* in 1998.[32] To calculate these costs, researchers Anne Wolf and Graham Colditz used the 1988 and 1994 National

> ***Nationally, the estimated annual cost attributable to obesity-related diseases is over $100 billion.***

Health Interview Surveys to determine the prevalence of obesity-related diseases such as Type 2 diabetes, coronary heart disease, hypertension, gallbladder disease, osteoarthritis, and cancers of the colon, breast, and endometrium. For each disease, the total cost was divided into direct and indirect costs. Direct costs included prevention, diagnosis, and treatment. Indirect costs were comprised of the wages lost by people unable to work because of their illness or disability and the potential wages lost due to premature death.

According to Wolf and Colditz, the total cost of overweight and obesity to the U.S. economy in 1995 was $99.2 billion, with $51.6 billion in direct costs and $47.6 billion in indirect costs. Table 9 shows the 1995 estimates by disease. More recent calculations have put the total cost of obesity (direct and indirect) in the U.S. at $117 billion.[34]

Table 9

Total Costs of Obesity, United States, 1995

Diabetes (Type 2)
- Total: $63.1 billion
- Direct cost: $32.4 billion
- Indirect cost: $30.7 billion

Osteoarthritis
- Total: $17.2 billion
- Direct cost: $4.3 billion
- Indirect cost: $12.9 billion

Coronary heart disease
- $7.0 billion (direct cost)

Hypertension
- $3.2 billion (direct cost)

Colon cancer
- Total: $2.8 billion
- Direct cost: $1 billion
- Indirect cost: $1.8 billion

Postmenopausal breast cancer
- Total: $2.3 billion
- Direct cost: $840 million
- Indirect cost: $1.5 billion

Endometrial cancer
- Total: $790 million
- Direct cost: $286 million
- Indirect cost: $504 million

Source: Obesity Research, March 1998

Among children, the economic consequences of obesity have risen dramatically. CDC surveys show an increase in annual hospital costs related to childhood obesity from $35 million in the period 1979-1981 to $127 million in the period 1997-1999. The number of days spent in hospitals by 6-17 year-olds more than doubled from 152,000 to 310,000 over the same time periods.[35] (Table 10)

Because the U.S. government is currently bearing the majority of the costs of obesity and related illnesses, Wolf claims, "the government is going to get slam-dunked in future obesity costs if it doesn't address the problem now. As the population ages and the prevalence of obesity continues to rise, Medicare is going to be picking up the healthcare tab for these people."[36]

<table>
<tr><td colspan="3" align="center">Table 10</td></tr>
<tr><td colspan="3" align="center">**Annual Economic Burden of Obesity Among 6-17 Year-Olds**</td></tr>
</table>

	1979-1981	1997-1999
Obesity-associated annual hospital costs*	$35 million	$127 million
Obesity-associated annual hospital costs**	0.43%	1.70%
Number of obesity discharges**	0.36%	1.07%
Obesity-related diagnoses e.g. diabetes**	1.43%	2.36%
Obesity-related gallbladder diseases**	0.18%	0.59%
Obesity-related sleep apnea**	0.14%	0.75%
Total days of care associated with obesity (days)	152,000	310,000
Length of hospital stay: principal diagnosis of obesity	6.35 days	13.46 days
Length of hospital stay: secondary diagnosis of obesity	5.01 days	6.76 days

* Based on 2001 constant U.S. dollar value

** As a percentage of total relevant hospital figures

Source: CDC National Hospital Discharge Survey (NHDS)

Part 3. Psychological Consequences

Overweight and obese people frequently suffer from social stigmatization, discrimination, and poor body image. It should come as no surprise that common psychological problems associated with overweight and obesity range from low self esteem to anxiety, clinical depression, and impaired social functioning.[37, 38] While these consequences are serious regardless of age, it seems particularly tragic for children and adolescents to be forced to deal with the issues of "growing out" in addition to the many challenges of simply growing up.

Some people have equated the social stigmatization of the overweight and obese with racism, and have called for increased education to promote tolerance. There is also a movement to adopt the concept of "healthy at any weight," which seeks to eradicate the negative self-image associated with overweight and obesity, and teach people to love their bodies regardless of size.

> *Promoting acceptance of overweight would be necessary only if there were no effective method to prevent or cure it.*

While prejudice against any individual based on appearance is morally repugnant, equally offensive is the suggestion that the overweight and obese should desist from efforts to lose weight and simply learn to love and accept their bodies. The physical and economic consequences of overweight are far too dreadful to allow inaction. Additionally, promoting acceptance of overweight would be necessary only if there were no effective method to prevent or cure it.

4

WHAT YOU SHOULD KNOW

> "''Knowledge is power.''
> – *Francis Bacon*

Part 1: Nutrition

The American humorist and philosopher Will Rogers once claimed, "It isn't what we don't know that gives us trouble, it's what we know that ain't so." Nutrition is no exception to this rule.

Calories

A calorie is a unit of heat that measures the energy-producing potential of food. The word comes from the Spanish word *calor* which means "hot" or "heat." A gram of fat contains nine calories while a gram of protein or carbohydrate contains only four calories.

Because of this difference, when the low-fat diet was initially advocated in the United States, it was widely assumed that reducing intake of dietary fat would yield a reduction

> *In America, average daily calorie consumption increased 12 percent–or 300 calories–between 1985 and 2000.*

in overall caloric intake. Unfortunately, the evidence shows that the opposite occurred: When Americans started eating less fat, they more than compensated for the reduction in calories from fat by eating a lot more calories from carbohydrates. Information gathered by the Economic Research Service of the U.S. Department of Agriculture shows that between 1985 and 2000 average daily calorie consumption in the U.S. increased 12 percent. This represents an increase of 300 calories per day.[1]

Considering the recommendations of the Food Guide Pyramid (see page 50), this increase seems inevitable. After all, the base of the pyramid includes up to 11 servings of bread, rice, pasta, and cereal–the carbohydrates with the highest caloric content. As a result of this increase, by the mid 1990s, children were consuming 54.5 percent of their total energy intake from carbohydrates.[2]

Portion Sizes

Just as portion sizes of fast food meals have increased substantially in recent years, so have portion sizes of meals eaten at home. A study conducted by researchers at the University of North Carolina at Chapel Hill found that portion sizes of foods such as hamburgers, burritos, tacos, French fries, sodas, ice cream, pies, cookies, and salty snacks grew larger between the 1970s and the 1990s regardless of whether people ate in or dined out.[3] For example, although the U.S. Department of Agriculture considers two to three ounces of cooked lean meat to be a serving, this study revealed that the size of hamburgers made at home increased from 5.7 ounces in 1977 to 8.4 ounces–more than half a pound–in 1996.

Fat

In the 1970s, Americans began to develop a fear of fat that has persisted and increased ever since. Today there is probably no other nation on earth whose inhabitants are more fearful of fat. Tragically, there is also no other country with as many overweight citizens.

Science journalist Gary Taubes addressed this issue in a *New York Times Magazine* article entitled "What If It's All Been a Big Fat Lie?" The cover of the magazine featured a picture of a juicy steak and the caption, "What If Fat Doesn't Make You Fat?" Taubes notes that the United States has become highly polarized on the subject of excess weight. "On the one hand, we've been told with almost religious certainty by everyone from the Surgeon General on down... that obesity is caused by the excessive consumption of fat. On the other, we have...what scientists would call the alternative hypothesis: it's not the fat that makes us fat, but the carbohydrates."[4]

As Taubes points out, if the "alternative hypothesis" is true, the actual cause of overweight and obesity is not overconsumption of fat but overconsumption of carbohydrates. This hypothesis is supported by data from respected researchers like Walter Willett, chairman of the department of nutrition at the Harvard School of Public Health. The data collected by Willett and others strongly suggest that the low-fat diet has failed not only in clinical trials but also in the actual lives of millions of Americans who have followed its precepts for over two decades.

> *If the "alternative hypothesis" is true, the actual cause of overweight and obesity is not over-consumption of fat but overconsumption of carbohydrates.*

The Skinny on Fat

The failure of the low-fat movement to produce the intended results may be due in part to the failure to distinguish among the various types of fat. Those who advocate the consumption of dietary fat say that the lack of distinction between "good fats" and "bad fats" causes low-fat advocates to throw out the baby with the bathwater. To counter this trend, diets like the Zone, Atkins, and Sugar Busters include varying levels of fat intake and generally claim that consuming certain types of fat has the following benefits:

> *The lack of distinction between "good fats" and "bad fats" causes low-fat advocates to throw out the baby with the bathwater.*

- Slows absorption of carbohydrates

- Produces satiety–the sensation of being full and satisfied

- Facilitates the absorption of vitamins and the production of hormones

- Does not stimulate production of insulin

Because all fats are not alike, it is important to understand the differences among the major fat groups: saturated, trans, monounsaturated, and polyunsaturated.

- Saturated fat is found primarily in animal protein, dairy products, and fried foods (French fries, fried chicken, etc.).

- Trans fats are produced artificially when polyunsaturated vegetable fats are hydrogenated, a process that increases both their firmness and their resistance to spoilage. Trans fat is commonly found in margarine, as well as many items labeled "low fat" or "reduced fat," such as crackers, chips, and cookies.

- Monounsaturated fats are found in certain oils (olive, canola, and peanut), nuts (pecans, almonds, cashews, peanuts, and walnuts), olives, and avocados.

- Polyunsaturated fats are commonly found in cold water fish (such as salmon), corn oil, safflower oil, soybeans, and flaxseed.

Bad Fat

Both saturated fats and trans fats are full of hydrogen atoms, which make them solid at room temperature. Because they are also solid at body temperature, these fats make it more difficult for the liver to absorb or filter harmful low-density lipoprotein (LDL) cholesterol, which is believed to clog arteries. Many experts assert that certain amounts of saturated fat can safely be included in the diet, but most suggest that trans fats be avoided entirely. Tragically, many of the foods recommended as healthy low-fat alternatives are loaded with trans fats. Examples include margarine, which the medical and nutritional establishment claimed would save us from heart disease and obesity, as well as many of the foods labeled "reduced fat" (check the label for the words "partially hydrogenated").

> *Many of the foods recommended as healthy low-fat alternatives are loaded with harmful trans fats.*

Good Fat

Most of the fats that have been proven to produce beneficial effects on the human body are mono-unsaturated. Because monounsaturated oils are liquid at room temperature and solids become liquid at body temperature, these fats make the liver membrane more "fluid" and allow cholesterol to pass more easily into the liver and out of the body. These fats have been shown to raise HDL (good) cholesterol and lower LDL (bad) cholesterol.[5] Additionally, monounsaturated fats make food taste better and make us feel full and satisfied, which helps us eat less.

Polyunsaturated fats, especially omega-3 fatty acids, have been shown to decrease both triglycerides[6] and the "stickiness" of platelets in the bloodstream.[7] One of the best sources of omega-3 fatty acids is cold water fish such as salmon and tuna. Unfortunately, because water pollution has contaminated some of the fish population, the risks of eating significant amounts of fish may outweigh the benefits. While farmed fish is less affected by pollution, the grain products in their feed may reduce the concentration of omega-3 fatty acids. Fortunately, the benefits of omega-3 fish oil can be obtained without the possible risk of consuming large quantities of fish by taking omega-3 fish oil supplements (capsules about the size of a multivitamin). Because the fish oils are molecularly distilled, contaminants such as mercury are extracted while the beneficial components are retained.

> *Eating proper amounts of the right fats has demonstrable health benefits. Consuming 30-40% of total calories from fat is considered reasonable by many experts as long as it is mostly monounsaturated.*

In conclusion, eating proper amounts of the right fats has demonstrable health benefits. Consuming 30-40 percent of total calories from fat is considered reasonable by many experts as long as it is mostly monounsaturated.

Carbohydrates

One of the more memorable aspects of the 1992 U.S. presidential race was the slogan "It's the economy, stupid." The purpose of this slogan was to focus attention on an issue that Democrats were convinced made President George H. W. Bush vulnerable. Today, a similarly energized group of Americans is seeking to unseat the incumbent low-fat diet by focusing on what they say is the real dietary cause of the national epidemic of overweight and obesity–carbohydrates.

Dr. Robert Atkins was one of the first widely-published experts to say that the admonitions against fat were ill-founded. His book *Dr. Atkins' Diet Revolution*, published in 1972, introduced a diet that was the opposite of what the government recommended. Contrary to the low-fat, high-carbohydrate American Heart Association diet, the Atkins diet allowed unlimited consumption of protein and fats but severely limited consumption of carbohydrates. Despite immediate denouncement of his diet by critics, Dr. Atkins sold millions of his books, which explained how to switch the body's metabolism from carbohydrate-burning mode to fat-burning mode by removing carbohydrates from the diet. While many nutritional experts have expressed concern about potential adverse effects of the Atkins diet, many scientists have concluded that Atkins was at least partially right about carbohydrates. Today, more than 30 years after publication of *Dr. Atkins' Diet Revolution*, scientists are exploring the benefits of a low-carbohydrate diet.

One such scientist is Dr. Walter Willett, chairman of the department of nutrition at the Harvard School of Public Health, who claimed "the pyramid really ignored 40 years of data and condemned all fats and oils."[8] He has also said, "the dietary pyramid was out of date the day it was printed, but it's even more out of date given the evidence that's accrued since that time."[9] Willett and other researchers believe that people who reduce body fat tend to do two things: increase "good fats" and "good carbohydrates" and decrease "bad fats" and "bad carbohydrates."

> **People who reduce body fat tend to do two things: increase "good fats" and "good carbohydrates" and decrease "bad fats" and "bad carbohydrates."**

Carbohydrates 101

To understand why some carbohydrates are considered "good" and others "bad," it is necessary to understand what carbohydrates are and how the body metabolizes them. One of the three building blocks of the diet, a carbohydrate is a nutrient consisting of carbon, hydrogen, and oxygen. Unlike the other two dietary components–fat and protein–all of the carbohydrates that are ingested are converted to glucose (sugar), which is transported to the bloodstream. In a sense, glucose is the human equivalent of gasoline–it is the fuel the body uses for energy. When glucose enters the bloodstream, the pancreas secretes insulin. When insulin is present in the bloodstream, the body burns carbohydrates for energy and stores the excess as fat to be used in the future. It is an elegant and wonderful design. The problem is that most of us:

1. Consume too many carbohydrates, which causes us to

2. Produce too much glucose, which

3. The body stores as fat, which

4. Is never burned as fuel, because

5. We keep eating more carbohydrates.

According to the advocates of the low-carbohydrate diet, to avoid this fattening cycle it is essential to eat only carbohydrates that do not cause the body to produce more glucose than it needs. For this reason, low-carbohydrate diets generally define "good carbohydrates" as those that do not cause an overproduction of glucose and "bad carbohydrates" as those that cause the body to produce more glucose than it needs.

The Glycemic Index

In technical terms, the degree to which any carbohydrate will cause a rise in the level of glucose when ingested is called its "glycemic index." The glycemic index is expressed as a number between 1 and 100 (the glycemic index of glucose). Foods with a high glycemic index produce a higher peak in blood glucose following a meal and a greater overall blood glucose response during the first two hours after consumption than do foods with a low glycemic index.[10] In other words, the higher the number, the more glucose that type of food will produce when ingested.

> **The higher the Glycemic Index, the more glucose that food will produce when ingested.**

Several large-scale studies from Harvard University indicate that the long-term consumption of a diet with a high glycemic load (glycemic index multiplied by dietary carbohydrate content) is a significant independent predictor of the risk of developing type 2 diabetes[11, 12] and cardiovascular disease.[13] Other studies indicate that a diet with a low glycemic load can protect against the development of obesity,[14, 15] colon cancer,[16] and breast cancer.[17] Finally, several studies have shown that the glycemic index is a good predictor of the concentrations of HDL (good) cholesterol in the healthy population.[18-20]

Bad Carbohydrates

Table 11 shows the most fattening carbohydrates (those with the highest GI), with the glycemic index of each food listed in parentheses.

Table 11

Most Fattening Carbohydrates
(Based on the Glycemic Index)

White foods	Other white flour products	Corn
• Bread (75-95)	• Pretzels (80)	• Kernel (60-75)
• Pasta (65)	• Cookies (55-70)	• Popcorn (55)
• Potatoes (95)	• Crackers (75)	• Chips (75)
• Rice (70-90)		

Source: American Journal of Clinical Nutrition

Breakfast Cereals

Most breakfast cereals are made from rice, corn, or refined wheat flour. Consequently, even cereals that are generally considered healthy have a high glycemic index, as evidenced by Table 12.

Table 12	
Glycemic Index of Certain Breakfast Cereals	
• Cheerios (74)	• Rice Chex (89)
• Cornflakes (92)	• Rice Crispies (82)
• Crispix (87)	• Shredded Wheat (83)
• Grapenuts (75±6)	• Special K (69±5)
• Raisin Bran (61±5)	• Total (76)
Source: American Journal of Clinical Nutrition	

Because many of the breakfast cereals preferred by children contain high concentrations of sugar and other sweeteners, it is not unusual for these items to have a glycemic index of 90 or higher.

Beverages

Many beverages contain carbohydrates and therefore have a glycemic index. Table 13 shows some high-glycemic beverages. Notice that beer has a glycemic index greater than 100. Beer contains maltose, a sugar produced in the brewing process that is actually sweeter than glucose. While most of us know that sugar-sweetened soft drinks are fattening, many mistakenly believe that fruit juice and sports drinks are better alternatives when in fact many of these beverages have an even higher glycemic index than soft drinks. The implication is clear: making water the beverage of choice can significantly decrease the glycemic load.

Table 13
Some High-Glycemic Beverages
• Beer (110)
• Cranberry Juice Cocktail (65-70)
• Soft Drinks, Sweetened (50–70)
• Sports Drinks (70-90)
Source: American Journal of Clinical Nutrition

Based on the glycemic index, it is apparent that many people who avoid dietary fat replace it with foods that are much more fattening. For example, look at Table 14, which provides a typical day's meals for someone trying to lose weight on a low-fat diet.

Table 14	
A Typical Low-Fat Diet for Adults	
Breakfast	Cereal with skim milk, toast with margarine and/or jelly; fruit juice
Lunch	Baked potato with margarine; yogurt
Afternoon snack	Pretzels
Dinner	Pasta, bread with margarine, fat-free cookies
Evening snack	Popcorn

Considering the glycemic index of these foods (see Tables 11-13), it is evident that in trying to control weight by restricting dietary fat, many people are consuming foods that produce the opposite effect.

Unfortunately, the diet of children and adolescents generally has an even higher glycemic load than that of adults. Many of the foods children prefer are high-glycemic items like pizza, macaroni and cheese, and French fries. Table 15 includes a typical weekday diet for a child.

Table 15	
A Typical Weekday Diet for Children	
Breakfast	Sugar-sweetened cereal, Pop-Tart®, fruit juice
Lunch	Peanut butter & jelly sandwich, potato chips, fruit snacks, fruit drink
Afternoon snack	Cookies, fruit drink
Dinner	Pasta, bread with margarine, ice cream
Evening snack	Popcorn or pretzels

Even more harmful is the weekend eating pattern for children. See Table 16.

Table 16	
A Typical Weekend Diet for Children	
Breakfast	Pancakes, waffles, or bagel
Lunch	Fast food: hamburger, French fries, soft drink
Dinner	Pizza, soft drink

Talk about a glycemic overload! The problem is that in following the low-fat recommendation, parents are allowing children a steady diet of foods that are likely to make them fat.

Breakfast Candy

Many American children begin their day with a glycemic overload in the form of breakfast cereal, breads, pastries, pancakes, waffles, and juice drinks. As shown previously (Table 12), breakfast cereals generally have a high glycemic index and, because most children's cereals are laced with high concentrations of sugar and other sweeteners, it is not unusual for them to have a glycemic index of 90-100. Table 17 shows other high-glycemic breakfast foods.

Table 17

High-Glycemic Breakfast Items
(Based on the Glycemic Index)

- Bagel, white (75)
- Cereal bar (60-80)
- Croissant (67)
- Doughnut (70-80)
- Pop-Tart (70)
- White bread (75-95)
- White flour, used in biscuits, pancakes, and waffles (70)

Source: American Journal of Clinical Nutrition

Lunch Candy

One measure on which the National School Lunch Program appears to be outperforming the alternative is in the amount of added sugars included in meals. Research shows that children who take their lunch to school consume nearly twice as much added sugar at lunch than those who participate in the school lunch program (22.9% vs. 13.2% respectively).[21] Many of the traditional lunchbox items consist mostly of high-glycemic carbohydrates. Table 18 gives some examples.

Table 18

High-Glycemic Lunchbox Items

• Cookies	• Peanut Butter
• Corn Chips	• Potato Chips
• Crackers	• Pudding
• Fruit Snacks	• White Bread
• Jello	• Yogurt
• Juice Drinks	

Source: American Journal of Clinical Nutrition

Good Carbohydrates

While some weight loss plans encourage dieters to avoid all carbohydrates, most experts recommend eating low-glycemic carbohydrates such as those shown in Table 19.

Table 19
Least Fattening Carbohydrates
(Based on Glycemic Index)

Green vegetables (glycemic index from 0 – 15)

- Asparagus
- Broccoli
- Brussels sprouts
- Cabbage
- Celery
- Collard greens
- Cucumbers
- Green beans
- Green peppers
- Lettuce
- Okra
- Peas
- Spinach
- Turnip greens
- Zucchini

Legumes

- Baked beans (40-50)
- Black beans (30)
- Black-eyed peas (40)
- Butter beans (30)
- Garbanzo beans (35)
- Kidney beans (30)
- Lentils (30)
- Lima beans (30)
- Pinto beans (40)
- Soybeans (15)

Fruit*

- Apples (30-40)
- Apricots, fresh (10)
- Apricots, dried (30)
- Banana (60)
- Cherries (25)
- Grapefruit (25)
- Grapes (50)
- Kiwi (50)
- Mango (50)
- Oranges (30-50)
- Peaches (40)
- Pears (45)
- Pineapple (65)
- Plantains (45)
- Plums (40)
- Raisins (65)
- Tomatoes (15)
- Watermelon (70)

Beverages

- Water (0)
- Apple Juice, unsweetened (40)
- Grapefruit Juice, unsweetened (48)
- Orange Juice, unsweetened (45-55)
- Tomato Juice, unsweetened (34-42)

[1]Because they contain natural sugars, some fruits such as watermelon, pineapple, raisins, and bananas have a higher glycemic index than green vegetables or legumes.

Source: American Journal of Clinical Nutrition

Protein

In the human body, protein is more plentiful than any other substance except water. Our muscles, skin, hair, nails, and eyes are all comprised primarily of protein. Of the 20 amino acids that form the building blocks of protein, nine are "essential amino acids" that cannot be synthesized by the body and must be supplied by diet. In short, we must consume protein to remain healthy. Table 20 supplies the current USDA recommendations for consumption of protein.

Table 20		
Recommended Dietary/Daily Allowance (RDA) of Protein		
	Age	**Amount**
Infants	Up to 12 months	13-14 grams
Children	1-3 yrs old	16 grams
	4-6 yrs old	24 grams
	9-10 yrs old	28 grams
Males	11-14 yrs old	45 grams
	15-18 yrs old	59 grams
	19-24 yrs old	58 grams
	25 and older	63 grams
Females	11-14 yrs old	46 grams
	15-18 yrs old	44 grams
	19-24 yrs old	46 grams
	25 and older	50 grams
Source: USDA Food and Nutrition Information Center		

Whole Grains

When the nutritional and medical establishment first started recommending a low-fat, high-carbohydrate diet, they may have assumed that Americans would mimic the diet of Asian countries such as China and Japan. In these countries, cooks spend considerable time shopping for ingredients and preparing meals. They also use a higher proportion of unprocessed or "whole" foods. It has been that way for thousands of years. In America, however, the focus is on speed and convenience. We want foods that can be purchased on the go or prepared in a matter of minutes.

Starting in the late 1970s, to meet the demand for foods that not only met these requirements but also adhered to the new low-fat standard, the American food industry began churning out baked goods such as bagels, muffins, and cookies, as well as quick-cooking items like pasta, minute rice, and frozen entrees. Unlike the foods consumed in Asia,

By the year 2000, Americans were consuming an average of 200 pounds per year of flour and cereal products, compared to 147 pounds per year in the 1980s and 135 pounds in the 1970s.

the new American foods contained highly processed ingredients. Because of this trend, the number of grain servings consumed by the average American jumped 33 percent between 1980 and

> *The problem with processed foods is that in order to make them more palatable or convenient, most of the fiber (and therefore the nutrients) are removed.*

2000, from 7.5 servings per person per day to 10 servings.[22] Grains (mostly refined ones) comprised nearly half of the increased consumption of calories during this period, compared to only 8 percent for fruits and vegetables.[23] By the year 2000, Americans were consuming an average of 200 pounds per year of flour and cereal products, compared to 147 pounds per year in the early 1980s and 135 pounds in the early 1970s.[24] In all, per capita consumption of total carbohydrates increased 21 percent between 1985 and 1999.[25]

The problem with processed foods is that in order to make them more palatable or convenient, most of the fiber (and therefore the nutrients) are removed. This results in products with high concentrations of what nutritionists call "empty calories." As a consequence of this trend, two-thirds of Americans are eating less than one serving of whole grains per day.[26]

In addition to their beneficial fiber content, whole grains are considered to provide several key health benefits, including:

- Important vitamins, minerals, and phyto-chemicals (plant substances such as flavonoids or carotenoids) that reduce the risk for some chronic diseases.

- A slow and steady effect on blood sugar and insulin levels that protects against heart disease and diabetes.

- Making us feel full (a condition known as "satiety"), which eliminates the unhealthy hunger pangs experienced after consuming a meal consisting of a large number of empty calories.

In the last ten years or so, scientists like Dr. Willett at the Harvard School of Nutrition have begun to understand that dietary fiber plays an important role in good nutrition. Dr. Willett conducted a study that showed dietary fiber intake is inversely correlated with heart attacks.[27] This helps to explain the results from Ancel Keys' Seven Countries study (Chapter Two), in which the countries with the highest rates of heart attack–the United States and Northern European countries–also had the lowest amount of fiber in the carbohydrates they consumed.

Nonetheless, many Americans are unaware of the health benefits of consuming whole grains. This ignorance may be due in part to the USDA Dietary

> *Many Americans are unaware of the health benefits of consuming whole grains.*

Guidelines, which suggest that all grains–whether whole or processed–are equal. (Although this problem was addressed in the 2000 edition of *Nutrition and Your Health: Dietary Guidelines for Americans*, which for the first time acknowledged the benefits of whole grains, this revision still failed to specify the number of servings to consume each day.[28]) Other reasons we do not consume many whole grain breads or pasta are that they are not readily available in restaurants or supermarkets, often take longer to prepare (brown rice, for example, takes twice as long to cook as white rice), and can be more expensive.

Table 21 lists the least fattening grain products (those with the lowest glycemic index).

Table 21
Least Fattening Grain Products
(Based on Glycemic Index)

- Brown rice (55)
- Oat or bran bread (50)
- Oatmeal (55)
- Rye bread (55)
- Sourdough bread (55)

- Whole grain pasta (40-45)
- Whole grain pumpernickel bread (50)
- Whole rice (50)
- Whole wheat pita bread (45)
- Wild rice (55)

Source: American Journal of Clinical Nutrition

Balanced Diet

By this point it should be clear that a healthy diet is none of the following:

- Low-fat
- High-fat
- Low-protein
- High-protein
- Low-carbohydrate
- High-carbohydrate

Instead, a healthy diet includes a consistent combination of:

- Lean protein
- Monounsaturated and polyunsaturated fat
- Low-glycemic carbohydrates such as green vegetables, legumes, and fruit

Shifting from a high-carbohydrate diet to a balanced diet generally involves getting rid of some foods and adding others. Tables 22-24 offer some guidelines to consider for making this adjustment.

Table 22
Guidelines for a Balanced Breakfast

Include	Exclude
• Butter	• Bagels
• Canola oil	• Biscuits
• Eggs or egg whites	• Cereal
• Fruit	• English muffins
• Lean meats (ham, turkey, Canadian bacon)	• Grits
• Nuts	• Jam, jelly, or preserves
• Oatmeal	• Margarine
• Olive oil	• Pancakes
• Whole grain bread	• Waffles
	• White bread

Table 23
Guidelines for a Balanced Lunch or Dinner

Include	Exclude
• Beans (black, green, red, navy, pinto, garbanzo)	• Corn
• Bread: whole grain, oat bran, rye, or pumpernickel	• Pasta
• Chicken salad	• Red potatoes
• Egg salad	• White bread
• Fish (salmon or tuna)	• White potatoes
• Green salad	• White rice
• Green vegetables	• Dessert
• Lean meat (ham, turkey, pork, chicken, beef)	
• Raw vegetables	
• Rice: brown or wild	
• Sweet potatoes	
• Tuna salad	

Table 24	
Guidelines for Nutritious Snacks	
Include	**Exclude**
• Berries	• Candy
• Cheese	• Chips
• Cold cuts (ham, turkey, roast beef)	• Cookies
	• Crackers
• Fruit	• Popcorn
• Hard boiled eggs	• Pretzels
• Nuts	
• Olives	
• Raw vegetables	

As we implemented these dietary changes in our household, my wife and I discovered an unexpected and liberating benefit: planning meals became much easier. Before we adopted the balanced diet, deciding what to prepare for dinner was an ordeal. Now it is amazingly simple. For example, here is a typical daily diet in the Hollander household.

Breakfast

- Scrambled eggs

- Fresh fruit

- Whole grain toast

- Turkey sausage or bacon

- Water or reduced-sugar orange juice

Lunch

The children pack a lunchbox with items from the top drawer of the refrigerator, which now contains only school lunch items, including:

- Zipper bags of lean turkey and ham. We simply roll up a few slices, stick them in the bag, and zip it up. Our kids prefer these "roll-ups" to a sandwich.

- String cheese. Mozzarella cheese sticks taste good and are an excellent source of protein and fat. This is also a wise choice for snacks at school or home.

- Whole fruit: Apples, oranges, grapes, peaches, pears, etc.

- Yogurt: Plain or low-sugar. We avoid the brands that come with a packet of candy or cereal to sprinkle in.

- Fruit cups: Mandarin oranges, peaches, or mixed fruit. Because these can be high in sugar, they should not be eaten every day but provide a reasonable substitute for fresh fruit or yogurt.

- Nuts. A handful of nuts makes an excellent dessert and wards off afternoon hunger pangs.

- Bottled water or sugar-free soft drinks.

Dinner

All we do is select a protein, two or three low-glycemic carbohydrates, and some healthy fat.

- Protein: Lean meat or fish

- Carbohydrates: Green vegetables, fruit, whole grain bread

- Fat: Olive oil for cooking and for bread (instead of butter); nuts for dessert

For our family, adopting this type of balanced diet has made food shopping and meal preparation far more simple. Although the children occasionally complain that our meals are monotonous, my wife and I are gladly willing to put up with a little grumbling because we know we are providing nutritious meals with a minimum of planning and stress.

SUMMARY

What You Should Know About Nutrition

- Dietary fat is good

- Monounsaturated and polyunsaturated fats are the best

- Trans fats are the worst

- Bad carbohydrates make us fat

- The worst carbohydrates are

  - White foods (potatoes, rice, pasta, bread, crackers)

  - Corn (including popcorn, chips, and tortillas)

- The best carbohydrates are

  - Green vegetables

  - Legumes

  - Fruit

- Sugar is bad

- The best beverage is water

Part 2: Exercise

"We are what we repeatedly do." — *Aristotle*

The evidence is undeniable. For people of any age, exercise improves health. Regular physical activity of at least moderate intensity has been proven to produce the following benefits.

Reduce the risk of:

- Heart attack
- Stroke
- Colon cancer
- Diabetes
- High blood pressure
- Coronary heart disease - the nation's leading cause of death
- Osteoporosis

> **For people of any age, exercise improves health.**

Decrease:

- Total blood cholesterol and triglycerides
- Muscle and joint pain
- Arthritis pain
- Stress
- Anxiety
- Depression

- Physician visits
- Hospitalizations
- The need for medications
- Falls among the elderly

Improve:

- High-density lipoproteins (HDL)-the "good" cholesterol
- Healthy bones, muscles, and joints
- Energy level
- Mobility
- Mental health

Components of Physical Fitness

A common way to approach physical fitness is to break it down into four components–flexibility, muscular strength, muscular endurance, and cardiorespiratory endurance. Here is a brief overview of each component.

1. **Flexibility:** The ability to move joints and use muscles through their full range of motion. The sit-and-reach test is a common measure of flexibility of the lower back and leg muscles.

2. **Muscular Strength:** The ability of a muscle to exert force for a brief period of time. Upper-body strength, for example, can be

measured by various weight-lifting exercises.

3. **Muscular Endurance:** The ability of a muscle or group of muscles to sustain repeated contractions or to continue applying force against a fixed object. Pushups and pullups are often used to test endurance of arm and shoulder muscles.

4. **Cardiorespiratory Endurance:** The body's ability over a sustained period of physical exertion to deliver oxygen and nutrients to tissues, and to remove waste. The ability to run or swim long distances are good indicators of this component.

A fifth item that is sometimes added to the list of fitness components is body composition. This refers to the makeup of the body in terms of lean mass (muscle, bone, vital tissue and organs) and fat mass. The ratio of fat to lean mass is an indication of fitness, and the right types of exercise help decrease body fat and increase or maintain muscle mass.

The F.I.T.T. Principle

A good way to ensure that an exercise program includes all the right elements is to use the F.I.T.T. Principle. This acronym outlines the key components of an effective exercise program:

F – Frequency (how often to exercise)

I - Intensity (how hard to exercise)

T - Time (how long to exercise)

T - Type (what kind of exercises to do)

The F.I.T.T. Principle is commonly used in the weight loss industry, and is also a part of many strength and weight training programs. The standard recommendation breaks down this way.

Frequency - 5 to 6 times per week

Intensity - Moderate to high

Time - 20 to 40 minutes per session

Type - A combination of cardiovascular and strength-building exercises

To better understand how the F.I.T.T. Principle can be used to achieve healthy weight loss, here is a closer look at each component.

Frequency

Many people are confused about how often to exercise. Most experts recommend some type of physical activity virtually every day, and suggest that cardiovascular exercise be performed three to five days per week. Those who are seriously unfit are counseled to start with less frequent exercise and build up over time.

Intensity

To monitor the intensity of exercise, many experts suggest measuring heart rate, either with a heart rate monitor or by self-calculation. To self-calculate, use a wrist watch with a second hand. Place your hand over your heart or feel for the pulse in your neck or wrist. Count the beats over a 15-second period and multiply by four. This yields the heart rate in beats per minute.

Some fitness experts recommend exercising within a "target heart range," which is simply a recommended range of heart rates measured in beats per minute. This advice is based on the assumption that heart rate accurately reflects the body's consumption of oxygen. Because this assumption is not always valid, some people who exercise in the target heart range may work too hard, while others may not work hard enough.

> *The goal of cardiovascular exercise is to get the heart, lungs, and muscles working well above the at-rest level and keep them there for 20-40 minutes.*

For most people, monitoring heart rate during exercise is probably unnecessary unless their physician recommends it. After all, the goal of cardiovascular exercise is to get the heart, lungs, and muscles working well above the at-rest level and keep them there for 20-40 minutes. Most people know their bodies well enough to recognize whether or not they are achieving this goal.

Time

While the duration can depend on the type of exercise, to improve cardiovascular fitness and reduce fat weight, most experts recommend at least 20-30 minutes of nonstop exercise most days of the week. For strength-building exercise such as weight training, sets and repetitions are more important than time spent.

> **Experts recommend at least 20-30 minutes of nonstop exercise most days of the week.**

Type

Like time, the type of exercise performed has a significant effect on the results. For cardiovascular fitness and fat loss, exercises such as walking, jogging, swimming, biking, stair climbing, aerobics and rowing are highly effective. To improve muscular strength, the most effective exercises include the use of free weights, machine weights, and body weight exercises such as pushups, pullups, dips, and Pilates.

SUMMARY

What You Should Know About Exercise

- Regardless of age, exercise improves health

- Fitness is a combination of

  - Flexibility

  - Muscular strength

  - Muscular endurance

  - Cardiorespiratory endurance

- Exercise is measured by

  - Frequency

  - Intensity

  - Time

  - Type

- Experts recommend at least 20-30 minutes of nonstop exercise most days of the week

Part 3: Weight Loss

Three Types of Weight Loss

To lose weight is to reduce the body's amount of water, muscle, or fat. Because only one type of weight loss appears to be desirable, it is important to understand the differences.

1. Water weight. The loss of water weight occurs constantly through the normal metabolic processes of perspiration and elimination. Losing excessive amounts of water weight results in dehydration. Because the body can store a lot of extra water, when a person increases physical activity it is common to increase both the amount of water consumed and the amount stored in the body. Consequently, an increase in activity can mask a reduction of fat or even produce an increase in total body weight.

   > *To lose weight is to reduce the body's amount of water, muscle, or fat.*

2. Muscle weight. This is weight that definitely should not be lost. Muscle weight is lost through either inactivity or a significant reduction in the number of calories

consumed. Because losing muscle weight produces the side effect of decreased metabolism, it is difficult to lose body weight by calorie restriction alone.

3. Fat weight. This is the weight to lose. It is a simple equation: If more calories are consumed than expended, the body stores the excess as fat. Fortunately, the reverse is also true: When the number of calories expended exceeds the number of calories consumed, the body breaks down fat to consume as energy. Since one pound of fat contains 3,500 calories, losing a pound of fat

> *The maximum possible fat loss for most people is two to three pounds per week.*

requires a 3,500 calorie deficit. Thus, to lose one pound of fat per week, one must create a deficit of 500 calories per day; to lose two pounds in a week requires a 1,000 calorie per day deficit; and to lose three pounds per week requires a 1,500 calorie per day deficit.

Because the maximum calorie deficit most people can achieve is 1,000-1,500 calories per day, the maximum possible fat loss for most people is two to three pounds per week. When a person loses more than three pounds in a week (a common claim of miracle diets) they may or may not have lost bad weight (fat), but have almost certainly lost good weight (water and muscle). Therefore, it is important to avoid regimens that promise rapid weight loss. Remember: Fat loss takes time.

Why Diets Fail

Calorie-restricted diets are usually unsuccessful for two reasons. First, when adults or children embark on severely calorie-restricted diets, no matter how much willpower they have, they eventually tire of never feeling full. Consequently, they get discouraged and either cheat or quit. Then they feel guilty for failing. This can be a demoralizing experience.

Second, many dieters find calorie-restricted regimens to be too complicated, requiring them to measure, calculate, and substitute various foods and dietary components. Other diets are too simplistic or rigid, allowing only one or two foods or types of food (the strawberry diet, the grapefruit diet, the all-juice diet, etc.). The reality is that we are unlikely to succeed with a diet that is hard to follow.

Third, calorie-restricted diets are often intended to produce only temporary results. The objective of many dieters is simply to shed excess weight and regain the freedom to

> *Calorie-restricted diets are often intended to produce only temporary results.*

overindulge. Thus, even those few people with enough willpower to endure the agony of extended self-denial find themselves in a vicious cycle of dieting and gaining weight.

Additional Weight Loss Principles

1. **Eating Less May Not Be Necessary.** For many people, changing *what* is eaten is more important than changing *how much* is eaten. This can be a liberating concept.

2. **Scales Are Unbalanced.** Because an increase in activity can produce an increase in stored water weight, the scale can be misleading. Since losing fat is a slow process, some children find the disappointment of weighing so discouraging that they are tempted to give up. Therefore, it is important for children to focus on their efforts-which should include a balanced diet and regular exercise-not on the results. Progress should be measured by factors other than weight.

3. **Exercise is Essential.** Healthy weight loss (i.e., fat loss) is a slow process that can only be achieved through a combination of diet and exercise. Fat is lost when more calories are burned than consumed. This requires fat-burning (aerobic) exercise. To increase the calorie deficit and prevent the body from consuming muscle rather than fat, one must engage in strength-building (anaerobic) exercises such as weightlifting, or body weight exercises (pushups, pullups, dips, Pilates, etc.).

SUMMARY

What You Should Know About Weight Loss

- There are three types of weight that can be lost:

  - Water

  - Muscle

  - Fat

- The only healthy way to lose weight is to lose fat

- The maximum amount of fat most people can lose is two to three pounds per week

- Calorie-restricted diets generally fail

- Eating less may not be necessary

- Weighing can be demotivating

- Exercise is essential

Conclusion

In his 2001 "Call to Action to Prevent and Decrease Overweight and Obesity," U.S. Surgeon General David Satcher wrote the following:

> *Many people believe that dealing with overweight and obesity is a personal responsibility. To some degree they are right, but it is also a community responsibility. When there are no safe, accessible places for children to play or adults to walk, jog, or ride a bike, that is a community responsibility. When school lunchrooms or office cafeterias do not provide healthy and appealing food choices, that is a community responsibility.... When we do not require daily physical education in our schools, that is also a community responsibility.*[29]

Dr. Satcher's focus on poor nutrition and lack of exercise as the cause of the current epidemic is laudable. His solution, however, slightly misses the mark. While there is undoubtedly a role for the community in solving this problem, the ultimate burden of responsibility should not be placed on the community. To do so is to subjugate our individual responsibility as parents, grandparents, educators, and caregivers to the bureaucracy, inefficiency, and personal agendas of others. In truth, we cannot beat this epidemic by committee. Instead, we must cure it one household at a time.

WHAT YOU SHOULD DO

"We must take responsibility both
as individuals and working together
to reduce the health toll associated
with obesity."
— *Tommy Thompson, U.S. Secretary
of Health & Human Services*

Overview

If your children are overweight, sedentary, or practicing
poor nutrition, here is good news: You can help them
develop a lifestyle of good nutrition and physical
fitness. The key word here is *lifestyle*. What children
need is not a crash diet or a boot-camp style exercise
program that gives them only short-term results.

Instead, they need to develop habits that will benefit them for the rest of their lives. The focus should be on the long term–not days or weeks, but months and years–and the time to start is NOW.

The First Five Steps

1. Acknowledge the problem
2. Accept responsibility
3. Examine yourself
4. Reprioritize
5. Develop a plan

Step 1: Acknowledge the problem

The first step in virtually any recovery program is to acknowledge the problem. Although it may be difficult or painful, you must admit that your child is sick. There are a number of reasons that you may be reluctant to make this admission. Here are a few.

Denial

A survey conducted by *Prevention* magazine revealed that many parents of obese children deny that their child has a weight problem. For those who do admit the problem, the tendency is to blame genetics. This study found that 46 percent of the parents of an obese child did not consider their child obese; 30 percent claimed that the obese child's diet was either healthy enough or as healthy as it could possibly be; and 46 percent believed that good health is determined predominantly by genetics rather than by diet and exercise.[1]

Pride

Although admitting there is something wrong with their children is difficult for many parents, for the sake of the children we must swallow our pride and acknowledge the problem.

Vulnerability

Examining the diet and exercise habits of children may leave parents, grandparents, and other adults feeling threatened that their own choices and behaviors will be subjected to scrutiny. This includes the possibility that they have used food (especially sweets) to endear themselves to children and reward them for good behavior.

Bad Advice

Over the last 25 years, millions of parents have unwittingly followed the erroneous advice of the nutritional establishment and served their children a diet of high-calorie, high-carbohydrate foods. As a result, children are not only consuming more calories per capita than their parents did at the same age, but are also eating a greater proportion of low-fiber "empty calories." A survey conducted by the American Obesity

Association showed that 44 percent of parents believed their children were eating more nutritiously than the parents did at the same age.[2] In addition to bad nutritional guidance, many parents have received bad advice from trusted

> *Parents may feel that solving their child's weight problem is simply beyond their capability. Take heart—it isn't.*

sources such as family members, friends, or even pediatricians, who have suggested that the child's weight problem was just "a phase" that would eventually be outgrown. Unfortunately, statistics show that overweight children are likely to become overweight adults.[3]

Hopelessness

Parents may feel that solving their child's weight problem is simply beyond their capability. Take heart—it isn't. Besides, we owe it to the children to give it our best shot.

Step 2: Accept Responsibility

There are two things for which we must accept responsibility. First, we must accept at least partial accountability for having created the problem. In all honesty, we have probably known for some time that our children have not been eating properly or getting enough exercise, but we have failed to take effective measures to solve the problem. This can be somewhat painful to accept. Maybe our priorities have been out of line. No doubt our intentions have been good. But one way or another, we have failed in our "prime

> *One way or another,*
> *we have failed in*
> *our "prime directive"*
> *as parents: to provide*
> *for the health*
> *and well-being*
> *of our children.*

directive" as parents: to provide for the health and well-being of our children. Although denial, pride, vulnerability, bad advice, and hopelessness are all valid explanations for creating or tolerating the environment and behaviors that promote childhood overweight, we must avoid making excuses. The truth is, allowing our children to become overweight or sedentary is a choice we have made.

Having accepted some responsibility for creating the problem, the next thing we must do is accept responsibility for *solving* it. Now is the time to drive a stake in the ground (that's stake, not steak), and take a stand for our children. Although you may be frustrated, avoid the temptation to throw open the window and shout: "I'm mad as hell, and I'm not gonna take it anymore." Instead, simply commit yourself to helping your child get well.

Notice that the commitment is not to *make* your child well but to *help*. This is a critical distinction.

Unless we hold our children under house arrest (which is not recommended), they will continue to have the freedom to make decisions about what they eat and how much they exercise. Thus, it is the

> *The most effective role for a parent in the child's recovery is not as a dictator but as a coach.*

child alone who ultimately must decide to eat right and exercise regularly. The most effective role for a parent in the child's recovery is not as a dictator but as a coach. As such, we should educate and encourage children to make good decisions even when we are not around.

Step 3: Examine Yourself

Answer the following questions honestly. Is your lifestyle setting a good example for your children? Do they see you exercise regularly and consistently eat the right foods? Do they know that you consider proper diet and exercise as important as bathing, brushing teeth, and cleaning their room? If you answered "yes" to each question, skip ahead to Step 4. If not, understand that before you can help your children get well, you must first get your own life in order. It's the old "physician heal thyself" thing.

Anyone who has flown a major airline in the last ten years has heard the safety instructions given prior to takeoff. You know the routine-a calm, pleasant voice says: "In the event of a sudden loss of cabin pressure, the oxygen masks located above the seats will drop down. If you are traveling with small children, place the oxygen mask over your own mouth and nose *before* assisting children with their masks." Although attending to their own safety before taking care of the children runs counter to the instincts of most parents, the reason for this advice is obvious: Parents who are dying cannot provide effective assistance to their children.

The same logic applies to diet and exercise. Before you can help your children, you have to get your own "oxygen mask" adjusted. To do this, you must formulate a plan for achieving proper nutrition and regular exercise in your own life. While this may not be the advice you were hoping for, consider the upside: This is a fabulous opportunity to initiate a discussion with your children. Here is an approach that has proven highly effective.

1. Get their attention. Tell them you have a problem with your health that you need to discuss with them.

2. Explain the problem. Tell them that as a result of poor choices you have made, you have increased your risk of heart disease, stroke, diabetes, and other deadly or debilitating diseases.

3. Ask for advice. Get their suggestions about how to change your habits and lifestyle to achieve a better diet and proper exercise.

4. Ask for help. Tell them you know it won't be easy and ask if they would be willing to support and encourage you.

As you engage your children in this process, remember this important principle:

> **For the next 30 days, make sure every discussion or activity related to nutrition and exercise is focused <u>100 percent on you</u> rather than on your children.**

There are three reasons for this. First, as a parent you need to lead by example. As with most of the important things we teach our children, it is not what we say but what we do that counts. One of the worst things a parent can say to a child is "do as I say, not as I do." If we are not practicing the behaviors we want to instill in our children, we have no credibility with them and will probably be dismissed as hypocrites.

Second, your child needs to see that you are serious-that this is not just a wish or passing fad. Have you ever fallen for one of those "get-fit-quick" schemes? Did you ever purchase a piece of exercise equipment and boast to your family how it was going to give you flat abs or bulging biceps, only to dust it off and sell it at a garage sale a couple of years later? Has your family ever seen you trying to shed excess weight on the grapefruit diet, the tomato diet, or some other form of foolishness? If so, when you

> *When your children see you losing weight and gaining energy and vitality, they may decide to change their own habits.*

announce that you are committing to proper nutrition and regular exercise, you should not be surprised or disappointed if your family members assume that this is just another get-fit-quick scheme. Only after seeing you practice what you preach will they be open to a conversation about themselves. After observing you for a period of 30 days, they should be convinced that you are in this for the long haul.

Finally, as you involve your family in the transformation of your habits and lifestyle, you give them ample opportunity to decide for themselves that they need to make changes in *their* lives. When your children see you losing weight and gaining energy and vitality, they may decide to change their own habits. This principle is a little like the front wheel drive car. Although cars were initially propelled from the rear axle, when manufacturers discovered that it is more efficient to pull a car than to push it, they switched to front-wheel drive. As we seek to change the behaviors of our loved ones, we should practice the front-wheel drive principle by pulling them along with us rather than pushing them into something new and different.

The fraction of an instant that children express a desire to start an exercise program or change their diet, we should extend an offer to help. However, it is critically important to resist the temptation to leap into action. If we are too assertive, they will probably feel that we are being pushy and will resist our assistance, no matter how well intentioned. It is equally important to avoid lecturing. To illustrate, consider two possible responses:

The Wrong Response

"Oh thank goodness! I have been so worried about you. You are so overweight and you never exercise. We are going to make some major changes around here."

The Right Response

"I think you have made a wise decision. I'm willing to help if you want me to. Is there anything I can do?"

Step 4: Reprioritize

Here is another painful fact. Lasting change cannot be achieved unless we adjust priorities and change behavior. The degree to which you and your children must change in order to develop a healthy lifestyle depends on the depth of the problem in your particular household. For some, the necessary changes in priorities and behaviors are relatively minor. For most, however, significant changes and sacrifices are required. For a few, radical action may be required to achieve the necessary changes (e.g., giving up a hobby, changing shifts, or even changing jobs). Because it is literally a matter of life and death, we must be willing to do whatever is necessary, even if this means changing our schedule, lifestyle, or even our income.

> *Because it is literally a matter of life and death, we must be willing to do whatever is necessary, even if this means changing our schedule, lifestyle, or even our income.*

Table 25 lists some priorities that may need to be changed and actions that may be required. As you review the list, in the left column circle or underline the priorities that need to be changed; in the right column, circle or underline the actions that must be taken. If you have additional suggestions you would like to share with others, please email them to:

wkoksuggest@worthypress.com

Table 25
Priorities and Actions for Nutritious Diet and Physical Fitness

Priorities	Actions
Eat meals at home	Get up earlier in the morning Leave work earlier in the evening Quit an activity Reschedule an activity Reduce fast food consumption
Eat meals together	Get up earlier in the morning Leave work earlier in the evening Quit an activity Reschedule an activity Change shifts Change jobs
Eat a nutritious breakfast	Get up earlier in the morning Eat at home Take breakfast to work or school Quit eating fast food Make or order a balanced breakfast (see Table 22)
Eat a nutritious lunch	Take lunch to work or school Eat at home Quit eating fast food Make or order a balanced lunch (see Table 23) Share meals in restaurants
Eat a nutritious dinner	Leave work earlier in the evening Quit an activity Reschedule an activity Eat at home Quit eating fast food Make or order a balanced dinner (see Table 23) Share meals in restaurants

Priorities	Actions
Reduce bad carbohydrates	Eliminate:
Increase good carbohydrates	Add:

Reduce bad carbohydrates

Eliminate:

-	Cake	-	Crackers	-	White bread
-	Cookies	-	Popcorn	-	White pasta
-	Corn	-	Potato chips	-	White potatoes
-	Corn chips	-	Pretzels	-	White rice

Increase good carbohydrates

Add:

Green vegetables

-	Asparagus	-	Collard Greens	-	Peas
-	Broccoli	-	Cucumbers	-	Spinach
-	Brussels sprouts	-	Green peppers	-	Turnip Greens
-	Cabbage	-	Lettuce	-	Zucchini
-	Celery	-	Okra		

Beans

-	Baked beans	-	Garbanzo beans	-	Lima beans
-	Black beans	-	Kidney beans	-	Pinto beans
-	Black-eyed peas	-	Lentils	-	Soybeans
-	Butter beans				

Fruit

-	Apples	-	Kiwi	-	Plantains		Eat sparingly
-	Apricots	-	Mango	-	Plums	-	Bananas
-	Cherries	-	Oranges	-	Tomatoes	-	Pineapple
-	Grapefruit	-	Peaches			-	Raisins
-	Grapes	-	Pears			-	Watermelon

Whole Grains   Bread

-	Brown rice	-	Oat
-	Oatmeal	-	Pumpernickel
-	Whole grain pasta	-	Rye
-	Whole rice	-	Whole grain
-	Wild rice	-	Whole wheat

Priorities	Actions
Exercise every day	Get up earlier in the morning
	Leave work earlier in the evening
	Quit an activity
	Reschedule an activity
	Change shifts
	Change jobs
	Purchase exercise equipment
	Walk or jog before breakfast
	Walk after breakfast
	Walk before lunch
	Walk after lunch
	Walk before dinner
	Walk after dinner
	Walk before bed
	Make walking a regular family activity
	Join a gym
	Take the stairs instead of the elevator or escalator
	Take fitness breaks at work by walking or doing desk exercises
	Get a push lawn mower instead of a riding mower
	Turn off the self-propel on your lawn mower
	Watch less television
	Videotape television programs that conflict with exercise times
	Exercise while watching TV
	Set a goal for steps or miles per day
Walk or ride a bike instead of driving	Walk when golfing rather than driving a cart
	Walk or bike to work, school, church, store, etc.
	Take the stairs instead of the elevator
	Park at the far end of the lot
	Get off the bus several blocks before your stop

Step 5: Develop a Plan

The more you plan, the more you increase the likelihood of success and decrease the time it will take to achieve results. Allowing children to make their own plans for exercise, meals, and snacks enables them to become eager and consistent participants. Conversely, if they perceive you as dictatorial and demanding, they are likely to resist.

As you develop your goals and plans, remember to be patient and realistic. Bear in mind that it took more than a few days or weeks to get to this unhealthy state and it will take more than a few days or weeks to get back to good health. Look at it

> *The more you plan, the more you increase the likelihood of success and decrease the time it will take to achieve results.*

logically: It is easier to gain weight than to lose it. So however long it took to gain the weight, it will probably take longer to lose it. It is a painful and unfortunate reality. To avoid disappointment, we must take the long-term view and bear in mind that the ultimate objective is not to lose weight but to develop healthy eating and exercise habits.

Plan Exercise

Developing an effective exercise schedule requires forethought and planning. Here are a few suggestions for making the planning process more effective and setting yourself up for success rather than failure and disappointment.

- Use an exercise diary to set goals and track progress. The diary in Appendix 2 can be downloaded free of charge from www.worthypress.com/wkok/diary.htm

- When setting goals, focus on the activity rather than the result. Setting goals related to frequency, intensity, time, and type of exercise is a recipe for success, while setting goals related to long-range benefits (weight loss, waistline, clothing size, etc.) is likely to produce disappointment.

- Use the Exercise Diary (either from the Appendix or the website) and the F.I.T.T. Principle (page 106) to plan the Frequency, Intensity, Time, and Type of exercise. Older children can do this on their own, while younger children may require assistance.

  - Frequency: Decide how many days per week to do fat-burning (cardiovascular) exercises, and how many days per week to do strength-building exercises (weight training or Pilates). Then decide which days of the week to perform each type of exercise.

- Intensity: For each workout, decide whether it will be moderate or intense.

- Time: Decide how long to perform each exercise.

- Type: Choose activities your children enjoy. To avoid boredom, choose several different types of exercises. Cross-training, as this is called, can also help prevent injuries caused by overusing certain muscles. Remember that both fat-burning and strength-building exercises are needed.

• Determine the best time of day to exercise. Is it early in the morning? After school? After dinner? Consider the child's schedule and energy level at different times of the day.

• Decide whether exercise will be done alone or with others. If your child revels in solitude, exercising alone can be just the ticket. However, an exercise partner may increase motivation or accountability. Exercise can also be a great family activity. For many children, a combination of solo and group exercise is most effective.

- Recognize your child's limits. Goals should depend on the level of fitness. For a child who is seriously overweight, a goal to run ten miles a day is not reasonable. A more realistic goal might be to walk briskly for 20 minutes. Remember to focus on the long term. It is important to set realistic goals, achieve them, then adjust them according to the new level of fitness.

- Seek support. It can help to tell friends about exercise plans and ask for their support.

- Include rewards. When setting exercise goals, decide on appropriate rewards for achieving them. This can be especially motivating for children.

- Educate your children. It is important for them to understand the importance of physical fitness. Discuss with them some of the data, principles, and recommendations in this book, including:

  - Overweight and obesity statistics (Chapter One).

  - The causes of childhood overweight (Chapter Two).

  - The consequences of overweight (Chapter Three).

- The F.I.T.T. Principle and the importance of both fat-burning and strength-building exercise (Chapter Four).

- The importance of setting goals and tracking progress (Chapter Five).

Plan Meals and Snacks

Planning what your children will eat can be as simple or elaborate as you wish. Some people like to plan a day or two at a time. Others prefer to plan an entire week or month of meals and snacks. Do whatever works best, but remember: Failure to plan meals and snacks can put your children in a dangerous

> *Failure to plan meals and snacks can put your children in a dangerous situation in which no nutritious foods are available.*

situation in which no nutritious foods are available. Making sure that healthy snacks like raw vegetables, fruit, cheese, and nuts are readily available at home and school will help your children avoid the siren call of junk food and vending machines. Similarly, thinking about where your children will be at mealtimes and what types of food will be available will help determine whether they should take a meal or snack.

As with exercise planning, it is important to involve children in planning what they will eat. The older children are, the more they can be involved and the more important it is to practice the front-wheel drive principle by pulling them rather than pushing them into better nutrition. This involves education. To avoid the sense that you are taking away their favorite foods, it is important to educate children to the extent that their age and maturity will allow. Discuss with them some of the data, principles, and recommendations in this book, including:

- The nutrition-related causes of childhood overweight and obesity, especially the Food Guide Pyramid, Fast Food, sugar, and the Children's Menu (Chapter Two).

- What they should know about fat, carbohydrates, and the glycemic index (Chapter Four).

- The importance of planning meals and snacks (Chapter Five).

Next Steps

At Home

1. Become a student of nutrition and exercise. There are many interesting and educational books, articles, and websites. The pubic library or local bookstore can help you get started.

Recommended reading

- *Eat, Drink and Be Healthy: The Harvard Medical School Guide to Healthy Eating* by Walter C. Willet, M.D.

- *The New Sugar Busters! Cut Sugar to Trim Fat* by H. Leighton Steward, et al.

- *The South Beach Diet : The Delicious, Doctor-Designed, Foolproof Plan for Fast and Healthy Weight Loss* by Arthur Agatston

Develop a habit of chatting with people who appear physically fit. Ask what foods and exercises work best for them.

2. Provide exercise equipment. Because children are not permitted in most gyms, they generally have limited access to exercise equipment such as treadmills, elliptical exercisers, free weights, or machine weights. If this is the case in your family, you may need to consider getting exercise equipment for your home. Although some equipment is quite expensive (especially treadmills), there are bargains to be had if you know where to look and what to look for. Consider used equipment from garage sales, flea markets, and classified ads.

3. Reduce Time with Television and Video Games

- Make a plan. Start by deciding how much time is appropriate for these activities. Make a list of alternate activities for the child's remaining free time.

- Communicate the plan. Discuss your concerns about the detrimental health effects of spending too much time watching television and playing video games. Explain the new rules and provide a list of alternative activities. Be positive.

- Use the When/Then technique: "*When* you have finished your homework and done your exercise, *then* you may watch TV or play a game." Establish this routine as standard practice.

- Expect Resistance. The most important job as a parent is not to make children happy but to ensure their wellbeing. The decision to limit time spent on these activities will not be popular. Expect great unhappiness. Be firm and loving, but stick to your guns.

- Change the schedule: If a child has a typical time for television or video games, such as after dinner, begin planning more activities during that time (e.g., a family walk).

At School

The most effective way to solve the problem of poor nutrition at school is to make sure that children leave home with a nutritious lunch consisting of a combination of protein, good fats, and low-glycemic carbohydrates. If taking lunch everyday is not feasible, at least check the school menu to see which days there will be food your child can eat. This does not mean that we should give up on the possibility that the school lunch program can be improved. To the contrary, we should dedicate ourselves to ensuring that the school cafeteria is providing nutritious meals. It is the right thing to do for the millions of schoolchildren who depend on this program for no-cost or reduced-cost lunches. However, we must accept that the problems with school nutrition will not be corrected overnight.

Here are some ways to work with the school to improve the quality of food and increase physical education.

1. Educate parents, teachers, and food service staff about proper nutrition, the importance of daily exercise, and the problem of childhood

overweight. Consider purchasing a copy of this book for the school library, principal, physical education instructor, etc.

2. Encourage parents and teachers to model good nutrition and regular exercise.

3. Suggest that the school district form a school nutrition advisory council comprised of parents, community and school officials, food service representatives, physicians, school nurses, dietitians, dentists, and other health care professionals. Offer to serve on the council.

4. Work to ensure that meals offered through the school breakfast and lunch programs contain a consistent balance of protein, healthy fats, and low-glycemic carbohydrates.

5. Suggest or support policies that:

   • Increase the prevalence of nutritious foods and beverages on school campuses.

   • Limit student access to vending machines and fast food.

   • Provide all children access to quality daily physical education and proper instruction in health education.

6. Support the recommendations of the "Soft Drinks in School" policy of the American Academy of Pediatrics,[4] which stipulates:

- Consumption or advertising of sweetened soft drinks within the classroom should be eliminated.

- School districts should invite public discussion before making any decision to create a vended food or drink contract.

- If a school district already has a soft drink contract in place, it should be tempered such that it does not promote overconsumption by students.

  - Soft drinks should not be sold as part of or in competition with the school lunch program, as stated in regulations of the US Department of Agriculture.

  - Vending machines should not be placed within the cafeteria space where lunch is sold. Their location in the school should be chosen by the school district, not the vending company.

  - Vending machines with foods of minimal nutritional value, including soft drinks, should be turned off during lunch hours and ideally during school hours.

- Vended soft drinks and fruit-flavored drinks should be eliminated in all elementary schools.

- Incentives based on the amount of soft drinks sold per student should not be included as part of exclusive contracts.

- Within the contract, the number of machines vending sweetened drinks should be limited. Schools should insist that alternative beverages be provided in preference over sweetened drinks in school vending machines.

- Schools should preferentially vend drinks that are sugar-free or low in sugar to lessen the risk of overweight.

At Restaurants

Solving the problem of poor nutrition at restaurants requires both a short-term and long-term strategy. In the short term, the most effective way to ensure that children eat nutritious meals in restaurants is to stop ordering from the Children's Menu. At most restaurants, there is little or nothing on the Children's Menu that children should eat.

If, like me, you are reluctant to pay the higher cost of an adult meal for a child, consider sharing. If you have more than one child, order a nutritious adult meal that they can share. If you have only one child, order a meal that the two of you can share. Because portion sizes have grown so large in recent years, my family (two adults and three children) often orders two entrees and one or two additional side items for the whole family to share. We save a lot of money this way and avoid overeating.

You can also reduce the caloric consumption of meals eaten in restaurants by drinking water or sugar-free drinks. To avoid the temptation to dig into the basket of bread when you are seated, try eating a handful of nuts or a piece of cheese before you leave home. Ordering a meal when you are ravenously hungry is dangerous. Finally, make it a habit to skip dessert.

The long term strategy is to insist that restaurants include more nutritious items on the children's menu, including smaller portions of grilled meat like beef, chicken, fish, and pork, as well as a selection of green vegetables.

Guidelines

Do

- Allow children to make decisions for themselves.

- Be a coach, not a drill sergeant.

- Be forgiving–there may be slip-ups and setbacks on the road to recovery.

- Be patient–losing fat and gaining physical fitness takes time.

- Be realistic–set reasonable goals and make reasonable plans.

- Be urgent–the time to start is now.

- Focus on foods that should be eaten, not those that shouldn't.

- Focus on health, not weight.

- Focus on what your children are doing well, not on what they aren't.

- Provide time for exercise after school.

- Praise good decisions.

- Become an advocate. Everywhere you go–work, church, neighborhood, social functions, etc.– look for opportunities to share what you have learned about nutrition and physical fitness (and of course, remember to mention this book).

Guidelines

Do Not

- Be a Hypocrite

- Deny hunger

- Focus on Weight

- Nag

SUMMARY

What You Should Do About Nutrition

- Reduce fattening carbohydrates

- Reduce sugar

- Provide a combination of protein, good fat, and low-glycemic carbohydrates

- Provide water instead of fruit drinks, soft drinks, and sports drinks

- Focus more on *what* is eaten than on *how much*

- At Home

  - Become a student of nutrition

  - Plan meals and snacks

- At School

  - Pack a nutritious lunch

  - Work to improve the lunch program

- In Restaurants:

  - Avoid the Children's Menu

  - Share

  - Skip bread and dessert

SUMMARY

What You Should Do About Exercise

- Tell your doctor or pediatrician that you are planning a regular exercise program. Ask if there is anything to be concerned about, such as monitoring heart rate.

- Engage in both fat-burning and strength-building activities

- Plan exercise

- Set goals and track progress

- At home:

  - Be willing to make sacrifices

  - Change priorities and actions

- At school:

  - Promote good nutrition and daily physical education

  - Offer to help

SUMMARY

What You Should Do About Weight Loss

- Provide balanced meals

- Exercise

- Focus more on *what* is eaten than on *how much*

- Focus on losing fat, not total body weight

- Weigh infrequently

- Be patient–weight loss takes time

CONCLUSION

"If we fail, at least let our children,
and our children's children say of us we
justified our brief moment here.
We did all that could be done."
— *President Ronald Reagan*

There is an epidemic wreaking havoc on America's children. The devastating effects are greater than those experienced by any previous generation. Left unchecked, the threat is as real and frightening as that of any terrorist group. Although our nation has declared war on international terrorism, we have failed to mount an organized defense against this epidemic of childhood overweight and obesity. In the conflict with this foe, there is no equivalent of the Department of Homeland Security.

The only way to defeat this enemy is by fighting house to house. All across America, mothers, fathers, grandparents, educators, and caregivers must take responsibility for helping children develop a lifestyle of physical fitness and good nutrition. To do anything less is to subject our children to the high probability of illness, disability, or premature death.

This battle can be won. The time to start is now. It is truly a matter of life and death.

Appendix A

Body Mass Index Diary

Name	Date	Height	Weight	BMI	Percentile	Date of Next Measurement	Goal for Next Measurement

This resource can be downloaded free of charge from
www.worthypress.com/wkok/diary.htm

Appendix B

Exercise Diary

Name _____   Month _____

Week 1	Sun	Mon	Tues	Wed	Thu	Fri	Sat
Goal							
Actual							

Week 2	Sun	Mon	Tues	Wed	Thu	Fri	Sat
Goal							
Actual							

Week 3	Sun	Mon	Tues	Wed	Thu	Fri	Sat
Goal							
Actual							

Week 4	Sun	Mon	Tues	Wed	Thu	Fri	Sat
Goal							
Actual							

Week 5	Sun	Mon	Tues	Wed	Thu	Fri	Sat
Goal							
Actual							

This resource can be downloaded free of charge from
www.worthypress.com/wkok/diary.htm

Introduction

1. American Academy of Pediatrics Committee on School Health. Soft drinks in schools. *Pediatrics.* 2004; 113(1):152-154.

2. American Obesity Association fact sheet. Obesity in youth. Internet: http://www.obesity.org/subs/fastfacts/obesity_youth.shtml. Accessed June 20, 2004.

3. Sears, B. *The Zone*: Revolutionary Life Plan to Put Your Body in Total Balance for Permanent Weight Loss. New York: Regan Books; 1995.

4. Steward, HL, Bethea, MC, Andrews, SS, and Balart, LA. *Sugar Busters! Cut Sugar to Trim Fat*. New York: Ballantine Books; 1998.

Chapter 1

1. National Obesity Education Initiative. *Clinical Guidelines on the Identification, Evaluation, and Treatment of Overweight and Obesity in Adults*. Bethesda, MD: National Heart, Lung, and Blood Institute; 1998. National Institutes of Health publication NIH 98-4083.

2. American Obesity Association fact sheet. Obesity in youth. Internet: http://www.obesity.org/subs/fastfacts/obesity_youth.shtml. Accessed June 20, 2004.

3. Centers for Disease Control and Prevention. Ten great public health achievements—United States, 1900-1999. *MMWR Morb Mortal Wkly Rep.* 1999;48(.12):241-243.

4. Centers for Disease Control and Prevention. Healthier mothers and babies. *MMWR Morb Mortal Wkly Rep.* 1999;48(38):849-858.

5. Ogden CL, Flegal KM, Carroll MD, Johnson CL. Prevalence and trends in overweight among US children and adolescents, 1999-2000. *JAMA* 2002;288(14):1728-1732.

6. U.S. Census Bureau American Fact Finder. Internet: http://factfinder.census.gov/servlet/DTTable?_bm=y&-geo_id=01000US&-ds_name=DEC_2000_SF1_U&-_lang=en&-mt_name=DEC_2000_SF1_U_PCT012&-_sse=on. Accessed June 20, 2004.

7. American Academy of Pediatrics Committee on School Health. Soft drinks in schools. *Pediatrics.* 2004; 113(1):152-154.

Chapter 2

1. U.S. Department of Transportation, Bureau of Transportation Statistics, NHTS 2001 Highlights Report, BTS03-05 (Washington, DC: 2003).

2. Nielsen Media Research, 2000

3. Annenberg Public Policy Center, Media in the Home 2000, p.7

4. Annenberg Public Policy Center, Media in the Home 2000, p.16

5. Annenberg Public Policy Center, Media in the Home 2000, p.19

6. Rideout, Victoria J. et al. ZERO TO SIX Electronic Media in the Lives of Infants, Toddlers and Preschoolers. The Henry J. Kaiser Family Foundation. Fall 2003

7. Crespo, Carlos J. DrPH, MS; Smit, Ellen, PhD; Troiano, Richard P., PhD, RD; Bartlett, Susan J., PhD; Macera, Caroline A., PhD; Andersen, Ross E., PhD (2001, March 15). Television watching, energy intake, and obesity in US children. Archives of Pediatric and Adolescent Medicine, 155, 360-365.

8. Dennison MD, Barbara A., Erb MS, Tara A., and Jenkins PhD, Paul L. (2002, June). Television viewing and television in bedroom associated with overweight risk among low-income preschool children. Pediatrics, 109, 1028-1035.

9. Jane E. Brody, "Metabolism May Make TV Fattening" Arizona Republic (April 5, 1992): p.L6

10. Ancel Keyes, et al, "The Biology of Human Starvation" (Minneapolis: University of Minnesota Press, 1950)

11. Keys A, Taylor HL, Blackburn H, Brozek J, Anderson JT, Simonson E. "Coronary heart disease among Minnesota business and professional men followed 15 years." Circulation 1963;28:381-95.

12. Keys A. Seven countries: a multivariate analysis of death and coronary heart disease. London: Harvard University Press, 1980.

13. Kannel WB, Dawber TR, Kagan A, Revorskie N, Sacks J. Factors of risk in the development of coronary heart disease: six year follow-up experience: the Framingham Study. Ann Intern Med. 1961;55:33–56.

14. Gordon T, Garcia-Palmieri MR, Kagan A, Kannel WB, Schiffman J. Differences in coronary heart disease in Framingham, Honolulu and Puerto Rico. J Chronic Dis. 1974;27:329–344

15. McGee D, T Gordon. The Framingham Study applied to four other U. S. based epidemiological studies of cardiovascular disease (Section No. 31). Bethesda, Md: US Department of Health, Education, and Welfare, NIH; 1976:76–1083.

16. Brand RJ, Rosenman RH, Scholtz RI. Multivariate prediction of coronary heart disease in the Western Collaborative Group Study compared to the findings of the Framingham Study. Circulation. 1976;53:348–355.

17. Multiple risk factor intervention trial. Risk factor changes and mortality results. Multiple Risk Factor Intervention Trial Research Group. JAMA. 1982 Sep 24; 248(12): 1465-77.

18. Taubes, Gary. "The Soft Science of Dietary Fat." Science, Volume 291, Number 5513, Issue of 30 Mar 2001, pp. 2536-2545.

19. U.S. Senate Select Committee on Nutrition and Human Needs. Dietary Goals for the United States, 2nd ed. Washington, DC, U.S. Government Printing Office, 1977.

20. Sears, Barry, Ph.D. Enter the Zone. Harper Collins, New York, NY, 1996.

21. David S. Ludwig. The Glycemic Index: Physiological Mechanisms Relating to Obesity, Diabetes, and Cardiovascular Disease, JAMA, May 2002; 287: 2414 - 2423.

22. Compiled by Economic Research Service, USDA, from NFCS 1977-78, NFCS 1987-88, CSFII 1989-91, and CSFII 1994-95, first-day intake data.

23. U.S. Department of Agriculture nationwide food consumption survey–What We Eat In America, 1995

24. Bureau of Labor Statistics. Consumer Expenditure Survey 1997

25. Putnam, Judy, Allshouse, Jane, Kantor, Linda Scott, "U.S. Per Capita Food Supply Trends," Food Review, Winter 2002, p.12.

26. Schlosser, Eric. Fast Food Nation: The Dark Side of the All-American Meal. Houghton Mifflin Co, Boston, MA, 2001

27. Shanthy A. Bowman, PhD, Steven L. Gortmaker, PhD, Cara B. Ebbeling, PhD, Mark A. Pereira, PhD and David S. Ludwig, MD, PhD. Effects of Fast-Food Consumption on Energy Intake and Diet Quality Among Children in a National Household Survey. PEDIATRICS Vol. 113 No. 1 January 2004, pp. 112-118

28. National Restaurant Association. Market-Driven Solutions. Internet: http://www.restaurant.org/pressroom/market_solutions.cfm. Accessed June 20, 2004.

29. U.S. Department of Agriculture (USDA), Food and Nutrition Service (FNS). National School Lunch Program Fact Sheet. Internet: http://www.fns.usda.gov/cnd/Lunch/AboutLunch/NSLPFactSheet.htm. Accessed June 20, 2004.

30. U.S. Department of Agriculture (USDA), Food and Nutrition Service. Children's Diets in the Mid-1990s: Dietary Intake and Its Relationship with School Meal Participation. January 2001, p. 128.

31. Centers for Dis ease Control and Prevention. School Health Policies and Programs Study (SHPPS) 2000

32. Henry T. Coca-cola rethinks school contracts. Bottlers asked to fall in line. USA Today. March 14, 2001:A01

33. Nestle M. Soft drink "pouring rights": marketing empty calories to children. Public Health Rep. 2000;115:308-319

34. Zorn RL. The great cola wars: how one district profits from the competition for vending machines. Am Sch Board J. 1999;186:31-33

35. Centers for Disease Control and Prevention. School Health Policies and Programs Study (SHPPS) 2000

36. Samuels & Associates, California High School Fast Food Survey: Findings and Recommendations. Public Health Institute, Berkeley, CA, February, 2000.

37. Pizza Hut. Nutrition Guide. Internet: http://www.yum.com/nutrition/documents/ph_nutrition.pdf. Accessed June 20, 2004.

38. The Coca-Cola Company. Your Health and Our Beverages: The Facts. Internet: http://www2.coca-cola.com/ourcompany/hal_facts_sedentary.html. Accessed June 20, 2004.

39. Pepsi Cola Company. Get Active, Stay Active. Internet: http://www.pepsi.com/help/getactive_stayactive/didyouknow/index.php. Accessed June 20, 2004.

40. American Academy of Pediatrics Committee on School Health. *Soft drinks in schools.* Pediatrics. 2004 Jan;113(1 Pt 1):152-4.

41. Centers for Disease Control and Prevention. School Health Policies and Programs Study (SHPPS) 2000

42. Youth Media Campaign Longitudinal Survey (YMCLS), Center for Disease Control, 2002

43. Youth Risk Behavior Surveillance (YRBS), Centers for Disease Control, 2002

44. HHS. Healthy People 2010, 2nd ed. With understanding and improving health and objectives for improving health. Washington (DC): GPO; 2000. 2 vol. p.22-19 through 22-23.

45. Andersen, R. E., Crespo, C.J., Bartlett, S. J., Cheskin, L. J., Pratt, M. (1998, March 25). Relationship of physical activity and television watching with body weight and level of fatness among children. Journal of the American Medical Association, 279, 938-942.

46. Putnam, Judy, Allshouse, Jane, Kantor, Linda Scott, "U.S. Per Capita Food Supply Trends," Food Review, Winter 2002, p.9

47. U.S. Department of Agriculture (USDA), Food and Nutrition Service. Children's Diets in the Mid-1990s: Dietary Intake and Its Relationship with School Meal Participation. January 2001, p. 66.

48. U.S. Department of Agriculture (USDA), Agricultural Research Service (ARS). Continuing Survey of Food Intakes by Individuals (CSFII) 1994-96.

49. Guthrie JF, Morton JF. Food sources of added sweeteners in the diets of Americans. J Am Diet Assoc. 2000;100:43-51

50. Calvadini C, Siega-Riz AM, Popkin BM. US adolescent food intake trends

from 1965 to 1996. Arch Dis Child. 2000;83:18-24

51. Gleason P, Suitor C. Children's Diets in the Mid-1990s: Dietary Intake and Its Relationship with School Meal Participation. Alexandria, VA: US Department of Agriculture, Food and Nutrition Service, Office of Analysis, Nutrition and Evaluation; 2001. Internet: http://www.fns.usda.gov/oane/menu/published/cnp/files/childiet.pdf. Accessed June 20, 2004.

52. Ludwig DS, Peterson KE, Gortmaker SL. Relation between consumption of sugar-sweetened drinks and childhood obesity: a prospective observational analysis. Lancet. 2001;357:505-508

53. Harnack L, Stang J, Story M. Soft drink consumption among US children and adolescents: nutritional consequences. J Am Diet Assoc. 1999;99:436-441

54. U.S. Food and Drug Administration, Code of Federal Regulations, Title 21, Volume 2 : 21CFR101.30 (Revised as of April 1, 2003)

55. Press Release: Brookdale Pediatrician Undertakes An Assessment Of Obesity In Children. Is Juice Abuse Contributing To Childhood Obesity? Brookdale University Hospital and Medical Center, May 19, 2003. Internet: http://www. brookdalehospital.org/html/news/news_051903.htm. Accessed June 20, 2004.

56. Colette Bouchez. "Fruit Juice a Two-Edged Sword for Kids," HealthScoutNews, May 5, 2003. Internet: http://www.healthday.com/view.cfm?id=513011. Accessed June 20, 2004.

57. Dennison BA, Rockwell HL, Baker SL. Excess fruit juice consumption by preschool-aged children is associated with short stature and obesity. Pediatrics. 1997;99:15-22

58. Mattes RD. Dietary compensation by humans for supplemental energy provided as ethanol or carbohydrates in fluids. Physiol Behav. 1996;59:179-187

59. Bellisle F, Rolland-Cachera M-F. How sugar-containing drinks might increase adiposity in children. Lancet. 2001;357:490-491

60. Tordoff MG, Alleva AM. Effect of drinking soda sweetened with aspartame or high-fructose corn syrup on food intake and body weight. Am J Clin Nutr. 1990;51:963-969

61. Coulston, Ann M. and Johnson, Rachel K. "Sugar and sugars: Myths and realities." Journal of the American Dietetic Association, March 2002

62. Dietz W. Health consequences of obesity in youth: childhood predictors of adult disease. Pediatrics. 1998;101:518-525

63. Whitaker RC, Wright JA, Pepe MS, Seidel KD, Dietz WH. Predicting obesity in young adulthood from childhood and parental obesity. N Engl J Med.1997; 337 :869 –873

Chapter 3

1. Allison DB, Fontaine KR, Manson JE, Stevens J, VanItallie TB. Annual deaths attributable to obesity in the United States. JAMA Oct 27;282(16):1530-8. 1999

2. American Academy of Pediatrics. Policy Statement: Prevention of Pediatric Overweight and Obesity. PEDIATRICS Vol. 112 No. 2 August 2003, pp. 424-430.

3. Gidding SS, Bao W, Srinivasan SR, Berenson GW. Effects of secular trends in obesity on coronary risk factors in children: the Bogalusa Heart Study. J Pediatr.1995; 127 :868 –874

4. Clarke WR, Woolson RF, Lauer RM. Changes in ponderosity and blood pressure in childhood: the Muscatine Study. Am J Epidemiol.1986; 124 :195 –206

5. Johnson AL, Cornoni JC, Cassel JC, Tyroler HA, Heyden S, Hames CG. Influence of race, sex and weight on blood pressure behavior in young adults. Am J Cardiol.1975; 35 :523 –530

6. Morrion JA, Laskerzewski PM, Rauh JL, et al. Lipids, lipoproteins, and sexual maturation during adolescence: the Princeton Maturation Study. Metabolism.1979; 28 :641 –649

7. Shinha R, Fisch G, Teague B, et al. Prevalence of impaired glucose tolerance among children and adolescents with marked obesity. N Engl J Med.2002; 346 :802 –810

8. Pinhas-Hamiel O, Dolan LM, Daniels SR, Standiford D, Khoury PR, Zeitler P. Increased incidence of non-insulin-dependent diabetes mellitus among adolescents. J Pediatr.1996; 128 :608 –615

9. Richards GE, Cavallo A, Meyer WJ III, et al. Obesity, acanthosis nigricans, insulin resistance, and hyperandrogenemia: pediatric perspective and natural history. J Pediatr.1985; 107 :893 –897

10. Must A, Spadano J, Coakley EH, Field AE, Colditz G, Dietz WH. The disease burden associated with overweight and obesity. JAMA. 1999;282:1523-1529.

11. American Academy of Pediatrics, Section on Pediatric Pulmonology, Subcommittee on Obstructive Sleep Apnea Syndrome. Clinical practice guideline: diagnosis and management of childhood obstructive sleep apnea syndrome. Pediatrics.2002; 109 :704 –712

12. Rodriguez MA, Winkleby MA, Ahn D, Sundquist J, Kraemer HC. Identification of population subgroups of children and adolescents with high asthma prevalence: findings from the Third National Health and Nutrition Examination Survey. Arch Pediatr Adolesc Med.2002; 156 :269 –275

13. Riley DJ, Santiago TV, Edelman NH. Complications of obesity-hypoventilation syndrome in childhood. Am J Dis Child.1976; 130 :671 –674

14. Boxer GH, Bauer AM, Miller BD. Obesity-hypoventilation in childhood. J Am Acad Child Adolesc Psychiatry.1988; 27 :552 –558

15. Mallory GB Jr, Fiser DH, Jackson R. Sleep-associated breathing disorders in obese children and adolescents. J Pediatr.1989; 115 :892 –897

16. Silvestri JM, Weese-Mayer DE, Bass MT, Kenny AS, Hauptman SA, Pearsall SM. Polysomnography in obese children with a history of sleep-associated breathing disorders. Pediatr Pulmonol.1993; 16 :124 –129

17. Dietz WH, Gross WL, Kirkpatrick JA Jr. Blount disease (tibia vara): another skeletal disorder associated with childhood obesity. J Pediatr.1982; 101 :735 –737

18. Loder RT, Aronson DD, Greenfield ML. The epidemiology of bilateral slipped capital femoral epiphysis. A study of children in Michigan. J Bone Joint Surg.1993; 75 :1141 –1147

19. Rashid M, Roberts EA. Nonalcoholic steatohepatitis in children. J Pediatr Gastroenterol Nutr.2000; 30 :48 –53

20. Squires, Sally (1998, November 3). Obesity-linked diabetes rising in children. Washington Post, pZ07, www.usda.gov/cnpp/ WP%20Obesity%20Article.htm

21. American Obesity Association fact sheet. Obesity in Youth. Internet: http://www.obesity.org/subs/fastfacts/obesity_youth.shtml.   Accessed June 20, 2004.

22. Dietz, William H., MD, PhD et al. Prevalence of a Metabolic Syndrome Phenotype in Adolescents. Arch Pediatr Adolesc Med. 2003;157:821-827.

23. American Heart Association. *Metabolic Syndrome*. Internet: http://www.americanheart.org/presenter.jhtml?identifier=4756. Accessed June 20, 2004.

24. Must A, Jacques PF, Dallal GE, Bajema CJ, Dietz WH. Long-term morbidity and mortality of overweight adolescents. A follow-up of the Harvard Growth Study of 1922 to 1935. N Engl J Med.1992; 327 :1350 –1355

25. Wisemandle W, Maynard LM, Guo SS, Siervogel RM. Childhood weight, stature, and body mass index among never overweight, early-onset overweight and late-onset overweight groups. Pediatrics.2000; 106(1)

26. Whitaker RC, Wright JA, Pepe MS, Seidel KD, Dietz WH. Predicting obesity in young adulthood from childhood and parental obesity. N Engl J Med.1997; 337 :869 –873

27. Guo SS, Chumlea WC. Tracking of body mass index in children in relation to overweight in adulthood. Am J Clin Nutr.1999; 70(suppl) :145S –148S

28. Calle EE, Thun MJ, Petrelli JM, Rodriguez C, Heath CW. Body mass index and mortality in a prospective cohort of U.S. adults. N Engl J Med 1999 Oct. 7;341(15):1097-105.

29. Stunkard AJ, Wadden TA. (Editors) Obesity: theory and therapy, Second Edition. New York: Raven Press, 1993, p. 224., National Institutes of Health. Clinical guidelines on the identification, evaluation, and treatment of overweight and obesity in adults. Bethesda, Maryland: Department of Health and Human Services, National Institutes of Health, National Heart, Lung, and Blood Institute, 1998, pp. 12-20.

30. Must A, Spadano J, Coakley EH, Field AE, Colditz G, Dietz WH. The disease burden associated with overweight and obesity. JAMA. 1999;282:1523-1529

31. Blumenthal D. Controlling health care expenditures. N Engl J Med. 2001;344:766-769

32. Wolf AM, Colditz GA. Current estimates of the economic cost of obesity in the United States. Obes Res.1998; 6 :97 –106

33. Finkelstein, Eric A., Fiebelkorn, Ian C., Wang, Guijing. State-Level Estimates of Annual Medical Expenditures Attributable to Obesity. Obesity Research January 2004.

34. Wolf AM, Colditz GA. Current estimates of the economic cost of obesity in the United States. Obesity Research 1998 Mar;6(2):97-106.)

35. Economic burden of obesity in youths ages 6 to 17 years, 1979-1999 Guijing Wang; William H. Dietz – Pediatrics May 2002

36. "The Growing Cost of Obesity, NACS Online, May 15, 2003

37. Strauss RS. Childhood obesity and self-esteem. Pediatrics.2000; 105(1)

38. Davison KK, Birch LL. Weight status, parent reaction, and self-concept in five-year-old girls. Pediatrics.2001; 107 :46 –53

Chapter 4

1. Putnam, Judy, Allshouse, Jane, Kantor, Linda Scott, "U.S. Per Capita Food Supply Trends," Food Review, Winter 2002, p.2

2. U.S. Department of Agriculture (USDA), Food and Nutrition Service. Children's Diets in the Mid-1990s: Dietary Intake and Its Relationship with School Meal Participation. January 2001, p. 66.

3. Samara Joy Nielsen and Barry M. Popkin, Patterns and Trends in Food Portion Sizes, 1977-1998. JAMA, Jan 2003; 289: 450 - 453.

4. What if It's All Been a Big Fat Lie?, Gary Taubes, New York Times, July 7, 2002

5. Kwiterovich PO Jr. The effect of dietary fat, antioxidants, and pro-oxidants on blood lipids, lipoproteins, and atherosclerosis. J Am Diet Assoc. 1997 Jul;97(7 Suppl):S31-41.

6. Sacks FM, Katan M. Randomized clinical trials on the effects of dietary fat and carbohydrate on plasma lipoproteins and cardiovascular disease. Am J Med. 2002 Dec 30;113 Suppl 9B:13S-24S.

7. Li D, Zhang H, Hsu-Hage BH, Wahlqvist ML, Sinclair AJ. The influence of fish, meat and polyunsaturated fat intakes on platelet phospholipid polyunsaturated fatty acids in male Melbourne Chinese and Caucasian. Eur J Clin Nutr. 2001 Dec;55(12):1036-42.

8. Carroll, Jill. "The Government's Food Pyramid Correlates to Obesity, Critics Say." Wall Street Journal, June 13, 2002.

9. The Low-Fat Legend: Is the Low-Fat, High-Carb Diet Mantra a Myth? ABC News, July 19, 2003

10. Kaye Foster-Powell, Susanna HA Holt and Janette C Brand-Miller. International table of glycemic index and glycemic load values: 2002. American Journal of Clinical Nutrition, Vol. 76, No. 1, 5-56, July 2002.

11. Salmeron J, Ascherio A, Rimm E, et al. Dietary fiber, glycemic load, and risk of NIDDM in men. Diabetes Care 1997;20:545–50.

12. Salmeron J, Manson J, Stampfer M, Colditz G, Wing A, Willett W. Dietary fiber, glycemic load, and risk of non-insulin-dependent diabetes mellitus in women. JAMA 1997;277:472–7.

13. Liu S, Willett W, Stampfer M, et al. A prospective study of dietary glycemic load, carbohydrate intake, and risk of coronary heart disease in US women. Am J Clin Nutr 2000;71:1455–61.

14. Ludwig D, Majzoub J, Al-Zahrani A, Dallal G, Blanco I, Roberts S. High glycemic index foods, overeating, and obesity. Pediatrics [serial online] 1999;103:e26. Internet: http://www.pediatrics.org/cgi/content/full/103/3/e26. Accessed June 20, 2004.

15. Ludwig D. Dietary glycemic index and obesity. J Nutr 2000;130: 280S–3S.

16. Franceschi S, Dal ML, Augustin L, et al. Dietary glycemic load and colorectal cancer risk. Ann Oncol 2001;12:173–8

17. Augustin L. Dietary glycemic index and glycemic load in breast cancer risk: a case control study. Ann Oncol (in press).

18. Ford E, Liu S. Glycemic index and serum high-density lipoprotein cholesterol concentration among US adults. Arch Intern Med 2001; 161:572–6.

19. Frost G, Leeds A, Dore C, Madeiros S, Brading S, Dornhorst A. Glycaemic

index as a determinant of serum HDL-cholesterol concentration. Lancet 1999;353:1045-8

20. Liu S, Manson J, Stampfer M, et al. Dietary glycemic load assessed by food-frequency questionnaire in relation to plasma high-density-lipoprotein cholesterol and fasting plasma triacylglycerols in postmenopausal women. Am J Clin Nutr 2001;73:560-6

21. U.S. Department of Agriculture (USDA), Food and Nutrition Service. Children's Diets in the Mid-1990s: Dietary Intake and Its Relationship with School Meal Participation. January 2001, p. 133.

22. Putnam, Judy, Allshouse, Jane, Kantor, Linda Scott, "U.S. Per Capita Food Supply Trends," Food Review, Winter 2002, p.4

23. Putnam, Judy, Allshouse, Jane, Kantor, Linda Scott, "U.S. Per Capita Food Supply Trends," Food Review, Winter 2002, p.2

24. Putnam, Judy, Allshouse, Jane, Kantor, Linda Scott, "U.S. Per Capita Food Supply Trends," Food Review, Winter 2002, pp.3-4

25. Putnam, Judy, Allshouse, Jane, Kantor, Linda Scott, "U.S. Per Capita Food Supply Trends," Food Review, Winter 2002, p.3

26. Putnam, Judy, Allshouse, Jane, Kantor, Linda Scott, "U.S. Per Capita Food Supply Trends," Food Review, Winter 2002, p.5

27. Bazzano LA, He J, Ogden LG, Loria CM, Whelton PK; National Health and Nutrition Examination Survey I Epidemiologic Follow-up Study. Dietary fiber intake and reduced risk of coronary heart disease in US men and women: the National Health and Nutrition Examination Survey I Epidemiologic Follow-up Study. Arch Intern Med. 2003 Sep 8;163(16):1897-904.

28. Nutrition and Your Health: Dietary Guidelines for Americans, USDA, 2000

29. U.S. Department of Health and Human Services. The Surgeon General's call to action to prevent and decrease overweight and obesity. [Rockville, MD]: U.S. Department of Health and Human Services, Public Health Service, Office of the Surgeon General; [2001]. Available from: US GPO, Washington.

Chapter 5

1. Prevention Magazine, 2003 Childhood Health Survey

2. American Obesity Association, Survey on Parents' Perceptions of their Children's' Weight, August 2000

3. Ogden CL, Carroll MD, Flegal KM. Epidemiologic trends in overweight and obesity. Endocrinol Metab Clin North Am. 2003 Dec;32(4):741-60, vii.

4. American Academy of Pediatrics, Soft Drinks in Schools. Pediatrics Volume 113, Number 1 January 2004, pp 152-154

Index

How to Order
We're Killing Our Kids

Internet

Purchase online at www.worthypress.com

Mail

Send check for $19.95 plus shipping ($4 for first book plus $1 for each additional copy; $10 outside the U.S.) Include your name, address, city, state, zip code, and email address. Mail to:

Worthy Press
P.O. Box 888685
Atlanta, GA 30356

ATTENTION CORPORATIONS, UNIVERSITIES, COLLEGES, AND PROFESSIONAL ORGANIZATIONS

Quantity discounts are available for bulk purchases of this book for educational or gift purposes, and as premiums for increasing subscriptions or renewals. Special books or book excerpts can also be created to fit specific needs. For information, please contact:

Worthy Press
P.O. Box 888685
Atlanta, GA 30356
sales@worthypress.com
866-809-3396